HERE IN THE NOW

AN ANTHOLOGY FOR THE SOUL

SHAI AFSAI   MARK ANDREW HEATHCOTE
CHRISTINE HERBSTRITT   MARYANNE J. KANE, PHD
MICHAEL P. KUSEN   SALLY QUON
K. V. RAGHUPATHI   WILLIAM JOHN ROSTRON
JIM TRITTEN

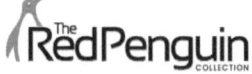

Hear in the Now–An Anthology for the Soul

Copyright © 2023 by JK Larkin

All rights reserved

Published by Red Penguin Books

Bellerose Village, New York

Library of Congress Control Number: 2023910910

ISBN

Print 978-1-63777-446-5

Digital 978-1-63777-445-8

No part of this book may be reproduced in any form or by any electronic or mechanical means, including information storage and retrieval systems, without written permission from the author, except for the use of brief quotations in a book review.

CONTENTS

ON FAITH Sally Quon	1
CAIN AND ABEL Maryanne J. Kane, PhD	5
THE KADDISH Shai Afsai	7
SAINT AGNES Michael P. Kusen	19
COMMUNITY ON 110TH STREET Michael P. Kusen	23
FINE SILK SPUN WITH GOLD Mark Heathcote	27
TOUCHED BY RAPTURE Jim Tritten	29
THE MINGO'S MESSAGE Michael P. Kusen	37
JEREMY'S SONG Christine Herbstritt	41
WHILE MY GUITAR GENTLY WEEPS William John Rostron	43
ORB OF LIGHT Mark Heathcote	53
SENSELESS William John Rostron	55
MANDOLIN MAN Michael P. Kusen	57
PRECIOUS TIME Mark Heathcote	61
THE ORDINARY MAN AND THE YOUNG PROFESSOR K. V. Raghupathi	63
About the Authors	85
Also from The Red Penguin Collection	89

ON FAITH
SALLY QUON

My mother was a teacher. As a young woman, she taught in a one-room schoolhouse in the country. She spent her life teaching, taking only a few years off when my brother, sister and I were young. I was in the fifth grade when she returned to teaching, first as a substitute and later as a full-time elementary school teacher.

When my mother passed away a few years ago, my brother gave the eulogy. He spoke about her love of teaching, how students would look her up, years later, to tell her how much of an effect she had on their lives. I remember every night after dinner, she would sit in her favorite chair marking papers and creating her lesson plan for the following day before retiring for the night.

I smiled to myself listening to my brother talk about my mom's love of teaching. She certainly taught me a thing or two. In fact, one of the most important lessons she ever taught me, she taught right there in the basement of the very church in which her service was being held.

We didn't go to church on a regular basis. Sunday mornings were usually reserved for an hour-long drive out to the country to visit my father's many siblings. But on those Sundays we didn't make the journey, mom would drag us down to the Presbyterian Church on the corner.

I can't say for sure whether I was the catalyst for the lesson. It was near Christmas and the story of Jesus, Mary and Joseph was likely what started the whole thing. I was having a hard time understanding how Jesus could be the child of Mary and Joseph and also the son of God. I cornered our fledgling minister and precociously demanded to know how God was born. He mumbled something about infinity and black holes and fled the room.

The next week, my mom was in charge of Sunday School.

Our class was small. There were only four of us, including myself. Each of us was given a choice. We could take the candy cane that my mother offered, or we could choose to take a small paperclip box. The catch was that we had no way of knowing what was in the box. It might be something great. It might be something not-so-great. The box might be completely empty. My classmates all chose the candy cane. I chose to take a box, pointing at the one I wanted.

My mother handed me the box. All eyes were on me as I opened it. It was not empty.

Inside the box were three jelly beans, a tiny doll with moveable joints, and a shiny new quarter.

"Sometimes," my mother said, "you have to believe in something, even if you can't see it. That is what faith is about. We may not be able to see God or Heaven, but that doesn't mean that they don't exist."

She ended the lesson by passing out the rest of the treats. All my classmates got a little box, none of which were empty, and yes, I got a candy cane.

I'm not a religious person – too many Sundays visiting relatives instead of going to church, I guess. But I never forgot the lesson. I use it every day. Faith is not necessarily about God and Heaven.

Faith is believing in something without guarantees.

I believe in the inherent goodness of people. I believe that even the worst person has some good inside them. I believe that most people would rather help you than hurt you.

Maybe more importantly, faith is about believing in myself. It's about believing that I can hit whatever curveball life chooses to throw at me. It's about believing that I can overcome any obstacle. It's about believing that regardless of what came today, tomorrow will be better.

I have faith.

Do you?

CAIN AND ABEL
MARYANNE J. KANE, PHD

Cain and Abel – the ultimate tale of sibling rivalry and death – much like my story.

The rivalry started early, in fact, in utero. During the first trimester, Doctor recommended multifetal reduction. Also called fetal reduction. Also called selective pregnancy reduction. If injecting a needle into the abdomen or vagina seemed barbaric, Doctor suggested radio-frequency ablation: blasting electric currents through the umbilical cord, obstructing blood flow to one of the babies...um, fetuses. Doctor always stressed that at 10 weeks, fetuses were the accurate description of what was growing in the womb. "It's a safe procedure and the chances of problems are small," Doctor said. *Well, yeah safe for the Doctor shooting death into the womb.*

Thus, for their first battle both babies scored a tie. In six months, together they entered the world prematurely, one weighing 3 lbs., 4 oz., one weighing 1 lb., 9 oz. Bethany Ramsey, or Beth, came home first, thriving quickly, gaining weight with a perfectly proportioned little face: almond shaped eyes, sweet-heart lips, button nose, and a heap of raven black hair. Bertha Ramsey, or Bert, struggled, requiring a longer stay in the NICU complete with a neonatal resuscitation bed, an oxygen mask, a breathing tube, and an occasional injection of adrenalin. Bert's underdeveloped torso gave her a malnourished achondroplasia look. She had very little hair on her head, but a ton of soft body hair called 'lanugo.'

Until hearing the word 'fraternal,' Beth and Bert's twin-status surprised people. People longingly gazed at Beth with admiration; they gawked at Bert with pity. Growing up, Beth scored high socially in popularity, invites to parties, club memberships. Bert scored high academically in test grades, class rank, and scholarships for college. Later in life, people gravitated towards Bert, her quick wit and political savvy gave the allure of an up-and-coming mover and shaker on the local government board-of-directors. Beth's interests - fashion, Botox and celebrity news - appeared superficial.

Equality between the sisters existed in only one category: their father's love. Beth's beauty or Bert's intelligence didn't factor in father's over-indulging treatment, both were his cherished gifts, both pampered unconditionally. For competing sisters, they had to out-do each other for father's attention and approval. Immature? Yes. Unhealthy? Maybe. Common? Very.

For years, Beth and Bert fought over their father: *I'll take dad to the doctor, I'm bringing dad on vacation this summer, I'll buy dad's suit for the wedding.* The feud continued endlessly, until one rainy afternoon when a discussion of where father would spend Christmas turned especially nasty. Unhappy childhood memories contributed to the squall: *You let my bird out of the window, you killed my pet fish, you were conceded, you thought you were smarter than me. I'm bringing dad to my house for Christmas. No, I asked first. He's coming with me.*

Throughout the yelling, neither sister noticed the father putting his hand up to his chest, gulping for breath. They were still arguing when he slumped over in his recliner, dead from a heart attack.

As I said, Beth and Bert – the ultimate tale of sibling rivalry and death – a mother's story.

THE KADDISH
SHAI AFSAI

Snow had fallen since morning, leaving the roads useless by dusk, and was still falling heavily. The city's plow trucks — though deployed in full force to clear the streets, sow them with salt and sand, and pile snow into residential driveways — were helpless in the face of such a downfall. The surface of the city stood like the fluffy interior of an immense cloud.

Above the empty streets and sidewalks, the bare branches of maple and oak trees sagged beneath their white weight, while the ropey electrical wires suspended between utility poles groaned in the wind. Snug within their homes, children, teenagers, and teachers delighted in the knowledge that school would be cancelled the next day, or at least delayed.

At the back of Petach Tefilah's smaller sanctuary — the larger one upstairs was reserved for *Shabbos* and holiday services — Judah Cohen stood huddled with six others who had braved the storm by foot. It was his wife's *yahrzeit*.

These seven, like most of the synagogue's members, were elderly men who lived nearby, for whom attendance at the *shul* was part of a daily routine. You woke up, located your slippers, had a cup of coffee, and headed to prayers. And you reversed the order before going to bed, substituting tea or perhaps warm milk for the morning's beverage.

They were few, these old men, but managed to gather a morning and evening *minyan* on most weekdays, as well as on *Shabbos* and holidays. During the winter, though, several of them vacationed in Florida. Others, whether due to their own preference or because their wives forbade it, did not venture outside their homes on particularly cold, snowy nights. Occasionally they prayed at Petach Tefilah with fewer than ten.

Puddles of melted snow had formed by the boots of the seven congregants. Having shaken off the cold and finished *mincha*, they stood at the back of the sanctuary, huddled around a table piled with prayer books and worn volumes of Gemara, on which Judah had placed a bottle of vodka.

Seated before his rolodex in an adjoining office, the gabbai was making phone calls. It seemed unlikely he could assemble ten men. Several members were out of town, including the rabbi. Jews who went to the city's other Orthodox synagogues were sometimes summoned to Petach Tefilah to assist with the *minyan*, especially if a *yahrzeit* was involved, but this was a storm to keep even the most devout away.

"Izzi Greene says he is coming," the gabbai informed the waiting men when he returned to the sanctuary. "No one else can show."

"That is only nine," said Judah. "What about Schwartz? Maybe he could help."

"No answer. I left a message."

"Did you call Rabbi Westel?"

"On a night like this? With his health?"

For five decades, before finally retiring, Rabbi Leon Westel had headed Temple Kol Shalom, the city's sizeable Reform congregation. Over the years, as both he and the members of Petach Tefilah had aged, and as many of them began passing away with increased frequency, he had more than once been the tenth man at the synagogue.

Rabbi Westel lived little more than a block away. Still, to ask the rabbi to venture out on such an evening…

"If we need him, we need him," said Judah.

"To guard against thieves, use a dog, but it is the cat that keeps mice away," added Jacob Gelder. He was inclined to aphoristic pronouncements, the meaning and relevance of which were usually unapparent to his listeners and often uncertain even to himself.

"What are you blabbering about? Now it is dogs and cats?" shouted Morris Kupot.

Half a century of synagogue association had fostered in Kupot a deep aversion to Gelder's philosophical outbursts. Once, some ten years before, overwhelmed by irritation, he had even stooped to hiding Gelder's favorite book, Lewis Henry's *Five Thousand Quotations for All Occasions*, which Gelder kept perpetually beside his seat in the smaller sanctuary, the better to thumb through during services. As the book's absence seemed only to worsen Gelder's proverbial predilections, however, Kupot reluctantly restored it. The passing decade had not undone the damage resulting from Gelder's discovery during those weeks when the book went missing that he need not rely solely on external sources but could also craft his own dictums for all occasions.

"It is the cat that keeps mice away. The cat," Gelder reiterated.

Izzi Greene announced his own arrival as he entered the synagogue. "Greene is here! Whew! So cold outside." He rubbed his hands together, but paused upon noticing the vodka bottle beside the prayer books and volumes of Gemara. "Ah, good. Vodka." He reached for the bottle.

"You keep away from that until after *davening*!"

"With Greene this makes nine."

"We have no choice. Call Rabbi Westel."

The gabbai went to his office to summon the Reform rabbi.

Greene's attention drifted from the bottle back to his surroundings. "Rabbi Westel? Why? What for? Outside I ran into a young Yid looking for the *shul*," he said, turning toward the door. "We have a *minyan*."

A stocky youth in his early twenties entered the sanctuary. He opened the door hesitantly with one hand, and with the other put a shiny purple yarmulke on his head, the relic of a long-ago bar mitzvah celebration now left as a spare in the synagogue.

Relief coursed through the air like a bird returning for spring.

"*Kum arayn, kum arayn,*" Gelder beckoned.

"So we have a *minyan*!" Kupot shouted. "Judah can say kaddish. Someone tell Lenny not to bother Rabbi Westel."

All smiles, Judah shook hands with the youth. "It is good you came."

"Jonathan Singer," he introduced himself.

"After we have some vodka, warm you up a little, Jonathan," Greene said, his attention once more drifting toward the bottle. Then he turned to the others. "This boy needs to say kaddish too."

The gabbai was fetched from his office.

"I was about to drag an old rabbi into this storm. You are the tenth. You made the *minyan*," he told the boy. To Judah he said, "That Rabbi Westel is a trooper. In this weather he was going to come out and help us."

"He is no spring chicken, either. Eighty-five now."

"A good man. Always willing to help."

The men were happy. Judah was elated. They had succeeded in assembling a *minyan* after all.

"Are you talking about Rabbi Westel from Temple Kol Shalom?" the youth asked.

"Of course. Who else? He is a true scholar. Studied in the Mir Yeshiva. Wrote books too."

"Very learned, in spite of being Reform. He translated the poems of Ibn Ezra."

"I know him!" the boy said. "He was at my circumcision. He taught me for my confirmation."

"Ha! You see? It is a small world with big men," declared Gelder, seizing the opportunity to indulge in an axiom. "People think it is the other way around, but no."

"It is also full of small men with big mouths, talking all the time about cats and dogs and birds and chickens," Kupot scoffed.

"Rabbi Westel even converted my mother," the youth continued. "And married my parents."

Judah looked nervously around, but no one else seemed to have heard. "Is that so?"

"How old is he now? Eighty-five, you said?"

Judah ignored the boy's question. "Did he convert your father too — Rabbi Westel?"

"No." A puddle of melted snow had formed by the boy's boots. "Just my mother. They met at college."

"Oh, at college. I see."

Judah and the gabbai's eyes met. Now all of the men realized there was a problem. They glanced at one another uncomfortably.

"I might need some help with the kaddish," the boy said.

No one responded.

"Who...who are you saying kaddish for?" the gabbai asked.

"My father. He passed away four years ago. Kol Shalom was closed, and I wasn't sure anyone would be here either with this snow, but I figured I'd give it a try. I saw your notice at The Cho-Zen about services every morning and every evening." He paused. "I had a bit of a hard time finding the place, though. You should get a neon sign out there." He chuckled at his own joke. "Good thing I ran into Mr. Greene."

Izzi Greene stared at the puddle beneath his boots. He felt somehow responsible for the situation. After all, he had been the one to encounter the boy outside the *shul* and bring him in.

The other men looked uneasily at one another, none sure what to do.

"It's lucky I found this place," the boy said. He checked his watch. "When do we start?"

Silence swayed in the sanctuary like white pines in a squall.

Gradually, the men's eyes settled on the gabbai. He saw to the day-to-day administration of the *shul*. They expected he would handle this matter too.

"We...we cannot have a *minyan*, son. I am sorry," the gabbai said.

Jonathan had begun to sense the room's unease. "Is it too late? I really wanted to say kaddish for my father."

"I am afraid it is now, yes. It is too late. You see, it is..." the gabbai began, but then stopped and sighed. "Come...come." He grasped the boy's hand and led him gently to the office.

Judah sat silently on a pew, disappointed and tired. He knew others who had sprung back from a spouse's loss to find new love, but for him it had been a vast melancholy of thirty years without his wife.

As happened often, and on every *yahrzeit*, memories of Rachelle's funeral swept over him. Nephews and cousins carrying her casket to the gravesite. Her remains slowly lowered into the cemetery ground. Shovel after shovel-full of earth piled on by neighbors and friends. When her casket was no longer visible, the grave almost full, he had crumbled. They had to hold him from either side while he said kaddish, the words as though coming out of another man's mouth.

∽

The gabbai gestured at a rusty metal folding chair.

"Please…sit."

The boy sat and the gabbai wheeled his desk chair over to him, close, so that their boots were almost touching. The gabbai rubbed his eyes with the backs of both hands.

"What's going on?" the boy asked.

"Too much. Too much is going on." The gabbai continued rubbing his eyes.

He had two grandsons about Jonathan's age, fine kids, handsome, though not as sturdy looking, not as solid or broad shouldered. Both grandchildren were in school. The older one was in graduate school, studying journalism part time, and worked as an usher at a Jewish funeral home. The younger one was in college and wanted to be a playwright — to invent plays for a living. Someone had allowed him to think this was a wise career choice. Probably his mother. But the boys' father, for his part, was not blameless either. He did not know how to be firm, their father. Worst of all, he had been lax with their religious upbringing. They could not read Rashi. A *blatt* of Gemara was like Chinese to them. They probably had not seen the inside of a *shul* since going off to college.

The gabbai looked at Jonathan. He seemed smart and sensible, a person studying chemistry or computers maybe, and not trying to be another William Shakespeare.

"How do I say this, Jonathan? Do you know what matrilineal descent is?" The gabbai did not wait for a reply. "This means we, Orthodox Jews, consider the religion of a child by the mother. You understand? The mother must be Jewish. A woman can convert, of course. Your mother converted. But she converted by Rabbi Westel. He converted her. We do not accept Reform conversions."

"I'm not sure I—"

Leaning forward, the gabbai took the youth's hand. "I do not mean to offend you in any way. You seem like a very nice boy. Not everyone would come say kaddish for his father, much less in a storm. You are a good son. I am only telling you how it is. For us, your mother is not Jewish and because of this—"

"My father was born Jewish. He never converted."

"Yes. But we go by the mother. I am sorry, Jonathan. We cannot count you for a *minyan*. Even though you are a nice boy, a good son, you are not Jewish."

Jonathan thought for a moment. "I don't know what you're talking about. I was born a Jew. I was raised a Jew. All my life I've been a Jew. My mother is Jewish."

"Not you or your mother. Not for us. I am sorry."

Jonathan avoided the gabbai's eyes, glancing instead around the office, at the rolodex beside the rotary phone, at the peeling paint and faded green carpet. He tried to work himself into a quick, justifiable rage, but the gabbai was still holding his hand, leaning toward him, and though he was hurt, Jonathan could not manage it.

Who were these people? he wondered. One minute they welcomed him, the next they wouldn't pray with him because his mother was a convert. They didn't look like the black-clad, bearded, medieval-minded Jews joked about at Kol Shalom, the Jews rumored to have sex through a hole in a sheet and to refuse to bury bodies with tattoos. But the centuries had skipped over these men all the same. They were breathing museum relics, ancient enough to warrant carbon dating. If they asked him to go, he would refuse. No one would prevent him from saying kaddish for his father.

"What now? Am I supposed to leave?"

"Of course not, Jonathan."

The gabbai was holding the boy's arm when they returned to the sanctuary. Jonathan was pale and shaken, and the eyes of both men were red. Although they had not yet prayed *maariv*, Izzi Greene opened the bottle and poured the vodka generously into plastic cups.

All ten took a cup and sat down in silence on the pews. Jonathan, asserting his right to remain, sipped his vodka too, feeling it burn in his stomach with each swallow.

The bottle was nearly empty and still no man had stirred from the sanctuary.

Worried women began ringing Petach Tefilah in search of their husbands. The wives of six of those present were still alive and nagging. Occasionally enlisting the support of a daughter or daughter-in-law, they reminded their husbands of the inclement weather and of the dangers of walking the dark streets on such a night. They foretold how their husbands might die of pneumonia contracted during the cold stroll home, if they did not crack their skulls on the slippery ice first, leaving the women lonely and destitute widows. With each call, Judah grew more despondent.

"I cannot stay much longer," Greene finally whispered. "It is not fair to Susie. Let us just *daven* without a *minyan*. We all need to get back home."

Judah turned to the gabbai. "Call Westel."

"It is late already. He might be sleeping."

"Good. Wake him up."

"When the sun has set, foxes walk by the light of the moon," Gelder said.

Kupot rolled his eyes. "This you already told us yesterday — foxes and the moon. It does not make any more sense tonight and it will not make any more sense tomorrow."

"Ah? You heard that one? I have to be careful then. When a dog starts chasing his tail, the weasel makes to steal the chickens."

The gabbai called Rabbi Westel, informing him that he was needed for the *minyan* after all. Rabbi Westel acquiesced immediately. The gabbai did not mention the boy.

Nearly half an hour elapsed before Rabbi Westel arrived — impeccably dressed, as for a wedding, but for his brown galoshes. He wore a black suit and tie, a starched white shirt with gold cufflinks. Leaning on his brass-topped cane, he looked frail but significant.

"You are a trooper, rabbi. Thank you for coming," said the gabbai.

Ever clever at math, the rabbi looked around the room and quickly calculated that ten men were already present in the synagogue.

Exhausted from the difficult walk and annoyed at having been unnecessarily troubled, he intended to promptly excuse himself and go home.

"*Rabbosai*, I am glad to assist, as you know. But the hour is late, and I am a tired old man, and seeing as you already have a *minyan*, I will retire to bed."

"We do not have a *minyan*," Judah said.

The rabbi counted once more. "You have ten here without me."

"We have no *minyan*."

Rabbi Westel noted the nearly empty bottle on the table and the plastic cups strewn about the sanctuary.

"This room stinks of vodka. Perhaps you are all a little too drunk to count?"

Reciting a biblical verse of ten words, he aimed an arthritic finger around the room, assigning a word to each of the congregants. "*Hoshia es amecha, uvarech es nachalasecha, urem venasem ad*" — he ended loudly with the boy — "*haolam*! There. With the young fellow, you have a *minyan*. I bid you good night."

"We have ten, yes. But we have no *minyan*, rabbi," Judah said, disappointment and anger in his voice. "You do not know this boy?"

Rabbi Westel looked at Jonathan, but could not place him. "Who are you, young fellow?"

The boy's voice cracked. "I'm Jonathan Singer, rabbi."

Rabbi Westel scanned the archival pages of his mind. "Jonathan? Marty and Katherine's son?"

The boy had filled out and grown since the rabbi had last seen him, become a man. Jonathan had been in the final confirmation class he had run at Temple Kol Shalom. By the time of his father's funeral, the rabbi had already been retired for a number of years, but he delivered a eulogy at Katherine's request. They had been such an attractive couple, Jonathan's parents, like French movie stars, the mother a lovely blonde, an utterly beautiful bride.

"You must stay, rabbi," said the gabbai, remaining near the boy.

"You see, Rabbi Westel, they don't consider me a Jew." Jonathan wanted to give full vent to his anger, to have it rise and be seen, but his voice emerged wounded and high-pitched. "I'm not enough of a Jew to count for their *minyan*."

"The rabbi can say kaddish for your father," the gabbai attempted.

"I'm his son! His son should say kaddish!" Jonathan was close to tears. "I'm a Jew!"

"Yes, but not to them," Rabbi Westel said.

"Look what you have done, Westel. Look what you have caused this boy and everyone here. Look!" Judah shook as he spoke.

"Me? I have caused? Who now refuses to accord this young man and his late father proper respect? Tell me. Who?"

"We cannot just pretend he is Jewish if he is not."

The rabbi struck the floor with his cane. "My conversions are real. He is not a Jew? Maybe I am not a Jew either?"

"No one said this, rabbi."

Rabbi Westel turned for the door.

He knew what Petach Tefilah's members thought of his denomination. On a personal level, they admired his erudition and scholarship and were grateful for his help with their *minyan*, yet his denomination lacked legitimacy in their eyes. Reform Judaism was to them nothing more than the one-hundred-and-fifty-year-old invention of *yekisher* assimilationists who, finding they lacked sufficient courage to convert to Christianity out and out and be done with it, had settled instead on making Judaism as close to a Protestant church as possible. Their physical descendants, however misled, were Jews — but who could accept their converts?

What did the men here make of his decision — him, raised and educated Orthodox, a former student of the Mir Yeshiva — to become a Reform rabbi? He thought of this often when he came to the *shul* and interacted with its members.

Perhaps, in their minds, it had been a career move rather than a philosophical or ideological one — his departure from Orthodoxy born of the desire to integrate more easily into America, and done for the benefits of prestige and salary connected to heading a large, well-to-do Reform congregation.

Every so often, surveying his life, he himself wondered if these had not been the actual reasons for his decision. Progressive and forward-looking though he was, he realized, he had never entirely shaken his *shtetl* roots.

But he felt that this sweeping dismissal tonight of the beliefs by

THE KADDISH

which he had chosen to lead his life and his congregation, this rejection of his right to oversee conversions, this refusal to count Jonathan for the *minyan*, were too much.

He addressed himself to the room. "The times change, and you all go on thinking like you are still in Europe."

The rabbi pushed open the door.

"Wait," the gabbai called. "What is the good in marching off? You walk out, we have no *minyan*. No one will say kaddish. Not Judah, not Jonathan. If you stay, Jonathan and Judah can say kaddish together. It is the only way."

"After this he asks me to stay," the rabbi grumbled. "After such insults they want me to make a *minyan*. Of what use are these prayers without knowing how to act toward one another?"

But he did not leave the synagogue.

"You have not missed a kaddish in the thirty years since Rachelle was *niftar*, Judah. You show the boy. Help him say kaddish for his father." Firmly holding a hand of each, the gabbai stood between the two and brought them together. "Jonathan, he will help you."

Judah opened a *siddur* and handed it to Jonathan as the gabbai donned a *tallis* and began intoning the evening prayers.

Rabbi Westel, standing by the now-closed door, prepared to answer amen.

SAINT AGNES
MICHAEL P. KUSEN

"I don't want it. What do I need it for?"

I leaned forward in my chair. "Mom, it's part of the package – the company just wants to make an appointment, to take a measurement, so the mold will fit properly."

Mom sat at the edge of her bed and gave me a smirk, "I walk fine with my friend here." She tapped her fingers on her metal prosthetic just below her right knee.

I looked down at the bright stainless-steel rod below the hemline of her housedress. "Mom, here look at this." I said holding out the brochure. "It's just a flesh colored mold to look like a normal leg."

"Normal? Normal is a real leg – this is not normal," she said lifting her prosthetic and jutting it out. "But it's fine with me. I don't care who sees it. I'm not hiding anything."

"It's not that you're hiding anything."

"Hiding things is for when you're ashamed of something!"

"It's just that it looks nicer because you don't wear pants so when you walk around

here that shiny silver rod looks like some kind of weird robotic part of you."

"And this I get from Captain Kirk? Looks nicer for who – a boyfriend maybe at eighty-two?"

My sister Alice stepped closer to mom pointing to her prosthetic, "Mom you look like a pirate with that leg."

"Well then maybe a swashbuckler will sweep me off my... foot!"

Alice clasped her hand as if to pray while rolling her eyes. I smiled and almost laughed at my mother twisting humor into her defiant stubbornness.

"Ok, forget it," I threw up my hands.

About a month later, I had a meeting with Sister Joan in her office concerning my mother's settling in at St. Saviors Nursing Home. Sister Joan stood up behind her desk, welcomed me in and invited me to have a seat in front of her. "Well, how is mom doing? Are you satisfied with the progress she's made adapting to being with us?"

"I'm very happy that she's here – everyone in my family is. St. Savior's is an excellent place for her to be. We could never care for her at home the way that you do. I think she's doing ok, but I know that it will still take time for her to accept all this."

"Yes, it often takes residents a few months to adjust to their new life with us."

"I just wish she wasn't so headstrong – sometimes she's a bit embarrassing."

Sister Joan looked at me with a quizzical smile. "What do you mean? How does she embarrass you?"

"It's not just me – it's the whole family. It's her prosthetic. She doesn't want to get the cosmetic covering for it – and she won't wear pants – so she walks around here like peg-leg-Pete – it's embarrassing."

Sister Joan's smile broadened, "I see." She closed my mother's folder on her desk and tilted her head down as she folded her hands together. She sat silent for a moment and then opened her hands as she started to speak. "I know that your mom is a strong woman – she's over eighty and walking on her own with her walker and *"peg-leg"* as you call it. Not many her age can do that – more often they sit in wheelchairs."

I shifted in my chair. "Yes, but people stare at her when she walks down the hall or in the lobby."

"Oh, I've noticed that too. In fact, some of the residents were a bit startled to see her at first."

"It's that shiny steel leg that scares them."

"Startles them, yes but I don't think it scares them. In fact, it wakes them up a bit."

"Wakes them up? What do you mean?"

"When they see your mom coming down the hall they see a very determined woman who is proud of overcoming her handicap – that's why she doesn't want to conceal it."

I slouched in my chair as the good sister continued.

"I saw the look on the residents faces the first time she walked into the lobby. Your mom and her leg got everyone's attention."

Sister Joan stood up and stepped over to the filing cabinet. She opened a drawer and pulled out a file. She opened it on the desk and took out a piece of paper and handed it to me. I looked at the poem that was written on it. "That poem was written by one of our residents, Florence. She used to write poems regularly for our monthly bulletin – then she became a bit despondent and stopped writing poetry. Then Florence befriended your mom and began writing poems again. Florence drew strength from your mom's example."

I sat up straight and listened intently.

"And she's not the only one of our residents who has been influenced by your mother. I've seen a few others who have perked up since she's been around. In an odd way, she inspires them. You know, God works in strange ways. Perhaps the good Lord sent your mom here to do his work through her." I sat silent thinking about what I just heard from the chief administrator of St. Savior's.

A short while later I was sitting on the bus on my way home wondering if they would eventually canonize my mom as Saint Agnes the patron saint of stainless steel.

COMMUNITY ON 110TH STREET
MICHAEL P. KUSEN

It was a late summer afternoon. Nancy would be seven next Saturday. She walked along the shore line in her pink and aquamarine bathing suit. Her feet played in the surf as her long brown ponytail swayed from side to side.

Labor Day had passed and Rockaway Beach was sparsely populated with plenty of open sand between the blankets. There were a few teenagers roughhousing in the water and some isolated bathers far down the beach towards 112th Street. It wasn't a very warm day but it was perfect for just relaxing listening to the rhythm of the surf and feeling the refreshing sea breezes. The beach widened at 110th Street. The boardwalk took a right angle turn at 109th Street, then corrected its direction after a few hundred yards, giving 110th Street a much broader beach area from the surf to the boardwalk. It was a favorite spot of many families being some distance from the younger crowd that congregated near 98th Street near the amusement park. The summer bungalows were close by so you got a mix of the local summer residents too.

Nancy's mother, Sharon, was directly behind the lifeguard stand about halfway between the stand and the boardwalk. She was changing her baby's diaper on the blanket. She powdered little Alex all up and changed his undershirt. Then she picked him up and laid him down in the port-a-crib. She glanced at her watch. It was three ten, and she knew that her husband Bob would be there soon to pick them up. She started gathering up her things, shaking out sand and putting them in her canvas beach bag. She stood up and looked towards the ocean. Cupping her hand above her eyes shielded out the sky's glare. Her petite and shapely figure was accented as she stood up on her toes to see further – but there was no sign of Nancy.

Thinking about what to do, Sharon turned and approached a white-haired woman who was sitting in a sand chair nearby. "Excuse me, would you do me a favor and watch my baby for a moment." She pointed to the port-a-crib. "While I… I have to go find my daughter."

"Sure honey. Go ahead" The woman got up and took hold of Sharon's hand. "Don't be nervous. I can see you're nervous. Go, go find your little girl. I'll watch the baby. Don't worry."

A few people watched Sharon as she walked rapidly over the hot sand to the ocean. She looked up and down the coast line but there was still no sign of Nancy. A few people stood up, detecting her nervousness. She ran back to the lifeguard stand. "My daughter is missing." She blurted out. "She was just here a few moments ago. I told her not to wander. We have to go soon. Just to stay in front of your stand down by the water."

"Ok." One of the life guards said as the other jumped down from the stand. "How old is she? What was she wearing?"

The other lifeguard on the stand extended his hand downward to Sharon. "Why don't you come up here and see if you can spot her along the beach from up here." Sharon grabbed his hand and climbed up onto the stand. "What does she look like?"

Sharon began to describe her daughter as they scanned the beach. Noticing Sharon on the lifeguard stand, a few people close by began to stand up and one man approached Sharon's blanket and started talking to the white-haired woman watching Alex. Nancy was nowhere in sight. The guard on the stand blew his whistle loudly as he relayed hand signals to the next lifeguard stand several hundred yards down the beach. In turn that guard stood, whistled and relayed to the next stand. Most of the people in the 110th Street area were now on their feet. Sharon was descending on the white wooden ladder with both lifeguards assisting her down the rungs.

"Look, here's what we're gonna do. Mark is signaling for a patrol car now. They'll be here in minutes. You said you had a picture of her in your wallet." Sharon's eyes moistened at the thought of her daughter's image. "Go get it. Wait by your blanket. I'll bring the cops over." There were six or seven people around the stand now.

"Don't worry we'll find her." A man's voice said as she walked back towards her blanket. A teenage girl in a bright yellow bikini walked by her side.

"Don't worry, she's got to be around here. I used to disappear around here all the time and drive my mom crazy when I was a kid." The girl lightly touched her hand to Sharon's shoulder as they walked.

When they reached her blanket there were several people gathered there. They were supportive with a chorus of words and gestures as she explained and described her daughter. Her shaking hands pulled Nancy's school photo from her wallet. The group took in the image of the young girl. Two men started walking swiftly towards the beach. Another made his way towards the boardwalk. Word of the missing child was being spread from blanket to blanket and a yellow bikini could be seen under the boardwalk weaving in and out between the support columns. "It's gonna be okay honey." The white-haired baby-sitter said, squeezing Sharon's hand.

"Here comes the cops." a masculine voice said as a patrol car came towards them riding on the boardwalk. Sharon looked up as they drove down the ramp onto the sand.

The baby cried and the white-hired woman picked baby Alex up and rocked him saying, "Now, now, Aunt Marie will take care of you." The baby settled down. The patrol car cruised on the sand and stopped as Sharon walked towards the car.

"My daughter's missing." She said holding out the picture. "She was just here moments ago." The cop on the driver's side examined the photo and began asking questions. Meanwhile the beach had turned into an area of little clusters of searchers and observers. In a few moments, the cops were gone with a promise to return shortly. She watched the patrol car ride down the beach. Calling out over their megaphone, "We are looking for a little lost girl whose name is Nancy." Sharon felt a shiver run through her at the sound of her daughter's name. The car slowly merged with other objects in the distance as its message faded.

At her blanket, she stood with strangers who were suddenly friends. She could feel their goodness. She stood taut, nervously erect as they conversed with her. One old man offered her some coffee from his thermos. Sharon took a deep breath as minutes passed that seemed to blur in her consciousness.

"I'm tellin' you, it's gonna be alright" Marie said, rocking the baby.

Sharon reached out for Marie's hand. "I hope. I hope. I ..."

"Are they comin' back?" She heard someone half-whisper from the edge of the crowd. Sharon turned her head abruptly towards the speaker and looked past him down the distant shoreline. She could see the patrol car in front of the ocean. It was slowly getting larger as she kept her eyes fixed on it. She felt her stomach churn and her shoulders stiffen as it came nearer. There was no megaphone message. The car veered on a diagonal heading straight toward Sharon.

"They're coming," the old man with the thermos said. Sharon felt numb as voices around her went mute and Sharon felt her heart pounding. She looked intently at the approaching patrol car. She stood frozen looking and squinting in the sun at the two figures in the car. She shielded her eyes with her hand recognizing the two patrolmen in the car. Then she saw a small head pop up from the back seat – and a wave of relief washed over her – suddenly there was salt air and a gush of warm blood and people talking, and Nancy.

"I told you it'd be alright" Marie said as Nancy got out of the police car. Nancy ran up to her mom and Sharon swept up her daughter into her arms. Nancy began chattering away as her mother squeezed her tightly. Sharon could let go of her tears now – not tears of sorrow but tears of joy. And all during the embrace, Nancy talked about the police car and the seahorse and the jellyfish and more as many smiles surrounded them.

Then slowly, like the receding tide, people began to disburse as 110th Street returned to its former state of isolated scatterings of people.

FINE SILK SPUN WITH GOLD

– Mark Heathcote

Folded moth wings placed together in prayer
open to discover the moon and starlit air
in madness flap, circle my heart
and like a curtain, take little bites at my soul.

But what can they discover - there!
My heart isn't threaded spun with gold.
And my soul isn't made of fine-silk
I'm just like the moon lost in this black ink.

With folded hands at night, I am locked-in sleep.
I dream and pray to fly away
indeed-there-are no limits to the madness I seek.
I even have the freedom to fly.

In madness flap, circle the light in a distant sky.
My prayers are never-more-spoken
as I draw back a curtain, which reveals a fine-silk
-spun with gold in madness, desires even my soul.

TOUCHED BY RAPTURE

JIM TRITTEN

JUNE 15TH, 2019, CORRALES, NEW MEXICO.

I turned my computer on, and after the screen settled down, I looked at a posting on Facebook. It was from an organization I had never heard of–No Barriers, USA. They were advertising openings for a nine-day Warrior expedition to Big Bend National Park in Texas. I scrolled down the page and saw it was open to veterans with a service-connected disability. The following motto permeated their website: "What's within you is stronger than what's in the way."

I watched a video about one of their co-founders, Eric Weihenmayer. Blind since his teenage years, Eric climbed Mount Everest. I thought, if he could do that, I could do this. I filled out the online application. After all, I had been a Navy carrier pilot and was used to meeting challenges on the fly.

On Saturday, October 5th, I joined nine other veterans and five leaders in Midland, Texas, for the most physically challenging experience of my life. We drove the next day to Big Bend, arriving around noon. We ate; then it got interesting. Humping it up a mountain with a pack almost did me in. I had to learn to accept and then ask for help from the young ones. That meant everyone else in the group. At the age of seventy-four, I was older than any of their fathers. One of the leaders wore a prosthetic leg – a souvenir of combat. Another participant had damage to both eyes and was legally blind. All the participants, including me, had a current diagnosis of post-traumatic stress syndrome.

I soon realized I was never going to complete the expedition without help. Accepting that I needed help was humbling, but the staff was very diplomatic in easing me through that barrier.

So I began to ask when I needed it and looked for opportunities to help others with the lessons age brings. And maybe even help somebody up when they fell.

Three days up, around, and down, the Chisos Mountain's beautiful wilderness fatigued every muscle in my body. Exhausted, I slept well on Tuesday night, October 8th, in the Rio Grande Village Campground. The next morning, I woke energized, ready for the next half of the expedition. I thought a bit of yoga would perhaps soothe my weary muscles and allow me to meditate about the experiences I had endured. And possibly contemplate the next four days, starting after breakfast, when we would travel thirty-three miles on the river in the canyons between Texas and Mexico, in kayaks.

At 6:30 AM, on Wednesday, October 9th, 2019, after freshening up, I remember starting my usual yoga practice. At some point, I lost immediate awareness of my position or how long I had held it. The last move I recall doing was the tree pose with my hands at the heart center. Then I felt the first salty tear. The tear slid down my right cheek and brought me back into semi-awareness. The most intense joyfulness filled every part of my being. An explosion of feeling like nothing I had ever experienced. Joy, pure joy. Beyond the intensity of holding my daughter for the first time. Way past the thrill of marrying Jasmine, the love of my life. An overwhelming merging of pure sensations and a mortal body accustomed to only slight variations of feelings – unless provoked. A perfect union of being present in the moment and an event with no beginning or end.

It was the most genuine experience of my life and the most exciting. I was at one with the universe. My eyes were open, but I could not see. I was outdoors and knew I was near a flock of birds noisily awakening from their night of rest, but I could no longer hear. I knew there were people cooking breakfast, but I could no longer smell. I could feel my emotions, but I could not feel my body touching the ground. No one could feel this great, I later thought. A happiness that brought tears to my eyes with no apparent trigger. Pure bliss. No separation of my physical body and the wild emotions uplifting my entire being. I remember smiling as the tears welled up in my eyes and fell on my shirt.

I have no idea how long the event lasted or how I got from the campground's fringes back to our group's site. "I think something just happened," I said as I looked at two of our leaders seated at a picnic table. They glanced up from their coffee cups and waited for me to say something more. "I can't explain what happened to me, but I'm going to give it a shot and say I feel like I've been reborn." I knew that wasn't the right phrase, but it was a start. I had generally given up on organized religion in my teen years and shuddered to think I had experienced some sort of religious reawakening. I walked away from the table and went into my tent and lay down.

At least I think I did.

I wasn't quite sure what to do about this "rebirthing" experience I had but knew the group was a safe place to express feelings and tell others what had happened. We shared our thoughts about the initial portion of the expedition at a campfire that first night on the Rio Grande. We repeated this sharing over the next few nights. We bonded as a group, and I focused on being grateful for the help, how challenged I was by the physical demands on my body, and for what had happened to me Wednesday morning in the campground.

Most of the vets gave me their thoughts about what happened. They made various suggestions either in a group setting around the campfire, or one-on-one with me. Some suggested it was Jesus talking to me. Perhaps I was being repaid with good karma for my hundreds of hours of volunteer work. I even thought maybe my then ninety-seven-year-old mother had let go and passed. No way to find out about the latter – we had no communications with the outside world. Plenty of time to reflect. In the end, I settled on a word I thought best described what happened to me – rapture. As I said the word rapture, I saw expressions of wonder on the other participants' faces.

Merriam-Webster defines rapture in the following ways:

1: an expression or manifestation of ecstasy or passion

2a: a state or experience of being carried away by overwhelming emotion

b: a mystical experience in which the spirit is exalted to a knowledge of divine things

3: often capitalized: the final assumption of Christians into heaven during the end-time according to Christian theology

Rapture–yes, that was the right word, even though I was not religious. I cannot recall ever using the phrase rapture verbally or in writing throughout my entire life. Having now consulted various sources on the meaning of the word, I accept the first two definitions and think it includes precisely what happened to me. But why me? Why now? And what was I supposed to do with it? I vowed to understand the experience and pledged to continue my investigation when I got back to civilization.

Who to tell and what to say to them ran through my mind as I rode in the van back to Midland. When we got into cell phone range, I texted Jasmine and told her I was still alive and would be headed home to Corrales the following day. I said nothing about the rapture, unsure how she would react.

The seven-hour drive home allowed me time to formulate what I wanted to tell Jasmine. I first recounted what happened during the nine-day expedition. I tiptoed into what happened on Wednesday morning, October 9th. Jasmine listened carefully and said that she knew something like that would happen. She added that she knew I had to take part in this expedition – she had never seen me so motivated to get myself into a semblance of good physical shape before I left for Big Bend.

I would not be satisfied until I had exhausted looking into all possible explanations of my experience. Why me? Why now? And what was I supposed to do with it? I sought out very close friends and family. I contacted a spiritual leader I knew who was extremely hard to reach but suddenly was available for a two-hour conversation by phone. I consulted my psychologist (who knows me inside out), nurses, doctors, a psychic, a minister, and my yoga teachers.

I went to my usual Thursday morning writing group at the Albuquerque VA hospital and met a young veteran who had never been there before. The young man started a discussion in which he recounted an experience he called an explosion of good feelings – being re-baptized. It could have been my story. He came to one more group session, and I have never seen him again.

People who I needed became available and were interested in my experience. All these people told me that what happened was not unique. It was unusual, but not unknown. Mystical events like this have happened to people all over the world for eons. One expert told me of the correlation between the body's and the mind's fatiguing and opening the body and mind to new experiences. Another said God is joy, and if I had experienced such an overwhelming feeling of pleasure… well, I was left to connect the dots myself. I started to think about all the Christian hymns and teachings that emphasize joy.

I did not post what happened on October 9th on my social media platforms. Only after some time passed, I started to open up to people I thought would accept my recounting of this story as truth without wondering if I had just flown in from a parallel universe. Those with whom I have shared my rapture experience have urged me to write about it.

∽

Let's address the questions I posed:

Why me? The short answer is because I answered an ad and decided with my right (intuitive) brain and pure gut instinct to participate in an intense, physically demanding expedition in the wilderness. Had I done a careful, time-consuming analysis of what I was going to face and understand the challenges ahead, I might have decided not to participate. But I acted instinctively and irrationally. An impulse guided me to join this trek without fully understanding the consequences. In retrospect, I'm glad I did, and I know I'm a better person for having done so. I have always trusted my instincts, and this time, some part of me understood why I needed to participate. My mind learned later.

Why now? Because I placed myself in a situation where I was in a new and pleasing physical environment, where I fatigued my body and made the switch to accept and even ask for help. I was open for something to happen to me on the morning of October 9th, 2019. I had worked for months to get ready for the expedition. For three days, I had been physically and emotionally challenged. My defensive walls were down, and I had been asking for and accepting help. I was surrounded by beautiful nature for an extended time. Equally important, I had no internet access. Instead, I was executing familiar yoga positions and meditating. Had each of these conditions not existed, the rapture might never have happened. It was like a perfect storm – just not at all threatening. Perhaps a higher power had heard me ask for help and answered in a way I could not possibly imagine.

What am I supposed to do with it? Why was this happening to me at the age of seventy-four? Then I replayed the mental recording of my fellow veterans who completed the experience. Each of them felt their own unique joy. I watched disabled veterans having fun, cannonballing with each other in the river. I empathized with returning soldiers acting like they were healthy. Perhaps my most memorable experience was following our legally blind Marine paddling his kayak down the river, in the lead, singing with his head bobbing from side to side like Ray Charles. Each veteran was touched by joy differently. That, too, gave me pleasure. I choke up every time I relive seeing these broken men and women happy. They gave all they could for our country and will forever pay the price for their service. They deserved joy and positive reinforcement.

We all have gifts. Mine include successfully flying off aircraft carriers, day or night, in the middle of the ocean with nowhere else to go. I was good at it and enjoyed being at the top of my game. My aviation career shaped my post-flying life. I rarely back down from a challenge, and I am glad for this expedition. I went with my gut. Navy pilots have an expression: kick the tires, light the fire, brief on guard. That's what I did – figured it out as I was doing it.

Another gift is my ability to put emotions and experiences on paper and create an effect in the mind's eye of a reader. Bottling up this experience is simply the wrong thing to do. There are messages from this experience for the reader. And I am supposed to share this experience with you. That is what I learned. Offering the event to readers or listeners with no expectation of anything other than to show joy was possible to me, a disabled vet, at the ripe old age of seventy-four.

No matter how bleak the circumstances, joy is possible in your life. Be open to receive it, and don't be afraid of taking a chance. Let down your defensive walls – but be in a safe environment when you do so. Not everything found on Facebook is right for you – but responding to this ad changed my life. Your joy may not occur in Texas, at a campground, or while doing yoga, but it may come to you in ways you would not anticipate. Staying at home, hunkered down, expecting the worst is not a likely path to experience joy or to receive unexpected healing.

I did not expect to find rapture when I went on this expedition. I don't think you can seek and discover rapture. It just happens. Rapture found me. My experience was a unity between a higher power and me. Perhaps nearing the supreme consciousness, or a peek at the Omega Point, envisaged by the Jesuit priest Pierre Teilhard de Chardin.

My rapture was brief, but it was real. My rapture was, without a doubt, the most unusual experience I have ever had. I passed the test. I performed well past what my logical brain would have said I was capable of doing. Who arranged for this test? I answered the ad, but I did not understand the degree to which I would be tested. Was it pure chance? Or was it part of a divine pattern designed to reveal itself in a way that would mean more than any sermon or words on a page?

I am forever grateful for having been challenged. For without that challenge, I might never have experienced what I did. Without that experience, I would not be telling this story.

And, with that story, perhaps you might think about truths that cannot be explained with the logical mind.

THE MINGO'S MESSAGE
MICHAEL P. KUSEN

The weeds were pushing up in Samuel Derring's front garden between the rainbow coleus, and the impatiens, between the daisies and the golden mums, in the rose bed and even through the pachysandra. Continuously they would resurge, gripping the earth to choke out weaker plants and grasses. It was their persistence that had worn Samuel down. Even stealing the pleasure he used to take in caring for his prized roses.

"Come on get yourself together" Samuel heard Bill's words echo in his mind, "You can start by pulling up these weeds." He sat on the white wrought iron bench which hugged the tall oak tree it arched around in the center of his garden. Toned by the shade of the oak leaves, his white hair was still bright with its handsome waves. His hands lay idle in his lap, thick, powerful and well-tanned.

Samuel closed his eyes, envisioning Bill's visit. He was sitting just as he was sitting now. The day was similar to today with light breezes. He saw the breeze parting the oak leaves causing sunlight to flash and strike at Bill as he paced along the garden's slate path. Bill was saying, "Sammy you can't be like this. You can't mope around here forever. This isn't you."

Samuel sat silent as his daydream continued

"This is nonsense." Bill stated with nervous assurance. "Plain nonsense. People have problems, tragedies even. You're not the only one. They get over them, and they go on. You know Jim Brokoff's kid was killed last Saturday – out in Oklahoma someplace. A car accident with his college buddies. He was the only one killed." Samuel watched his friend as he reached the end of the path, turned and came back towards him.

"I'm sorry." Samuel said in a low voice as Bill neared. "Tell Jim I'm sorry."

"You tell him. You tell him you're sorry." Bill shot back. "That is if you ever go down to the post again." Bill said, letting his nervousness get the best of him.

"I just don't feel like it."

"I know, I know, you don't feel like it." Bill stood directly before his friend. "It's been almost six weeks." He lowered his voice. "Now come to the meeting this week. We're making plans for the Memorial Day parade. You know the guys ask about you, and I feel like a jerk."

Samuel shifted in his seat.

"I'm your best friend. We grew up together. We went to war together for Christ sake."

"Look Bill" Samuel started.

"No, you look." Bill fired angrily. "I know Helen meant a lot to you. Nobody wants to lose their wife, Goddammit! But it happens. And it ends. And it's over. Time passes... enough already, you've got to live for you now. I mean, I feel like you're dragging me down in this thing you do, moping around here doing nothing."

Samuel's eyes widened as Bill's tensions oscillated. Bill pulled a handkerchief from his pocket, blew his nose and wiped moisture from the corner of his eyes as he stepped away. Then regaining his composure, he stepped forward leaning downward to be at eye level with Samuel sitting on the bench and put his hand on Samuel's shoulder. "Sammy, come down to the meeting this Friday, please Sammy for me. I'm countin'on ya." Bill's voice faded in Samuel's mind along with his image and the awkwardness he felt at that moment.

A faint sound caused Samuel to open his eyes. He saw a blonde curly haired toddler making his way up the entrance step and into his garden. The boy slowly panned from side to side as he walked, his large brown eyes absorbing the colors of the garden. He looked at Samuel in passing as though he were part of the foliage. Then his glance returned, as he gracefully tilted his head looking at Samuel with a new interest and announced, "I went to the zoo." The child was unfamiliar to Samuel. Not from our neighborhood he thought looking down the sidewalk for some sign of a parent. "I went to the zoo!" he repeated, demanding to be looked at.

"Where's your mommy?" Samuel responded to his little visitor.

"And I saw am-in-uls and mingos!" the boy continued as though Samuel had never asked a question. He stepped wobbly towards Samuel and put his hand on Samuel's knee to steady himself.

Through a faint smile Samuel asked softly, "Mingos huh, what are mingos?"

The little visitor stopped all movement at the question. Only his large brown eyes moving back and forth showed his concentration. Then he blurted out, "Pink, they pink."

A faint smile came to Samuel's lips at the description of the imaginary animal. "I've never seen that kind of an animal. Does he live at your house?"

The boy waved his hand up and down and then slid it into the pocket of his tan shorts.

He seemed to be searching for something as a quizzical expression came on to his little brow that made Samuel snicker. The little guy tugged on something in his pocket and yanked a wrinkled picture postcard. He held it down for a moment and then popped it up to Samuel saying, "Seeeeeee, mingos, mingos, mingos."

On the postcard was a group of flamingos standing in a lagoon. Samuel shook his head in acknowledgement and a faint smile broke into a chuckle.

"Michael" a woman's voice called from some distance. Samuel looked up and could see a young woman rapidly approaching from down the block.

"Michael," she cried again as she came closer.

Samuel's little visitor froze like a garden statue at the sound of his mother's voice.

"So, it's Michael is it?" Samuel inquired, as his little guest's face put on an impish, innocent look. A few moments later mother and son were walking away after some tender exchanges punctuated by an apologetic explanation to Samuel.

"No trouble at all." was Samuel's parting remark, "Your little guy was kind of enjoyable, and I learned about his mingos" Samuel eyes squinted as his smile broadened.

Alone in his garden again Samuel closed his eyes for a moment and when he opened them he saw his garden differently. He saw all the invading weeds among his flowers. Suddenly they irritated him. He rose up from the bench and went into the house. Moments later he returned and as he opened the door the sun reflected silver highlights from his white hair. His strong left hand gripped the handrail as he descended the front steps. In his right hand was a spade. He marched straight for the rose bed and vigorously thrust the spade into the dry earth. With his other hand he grabbed the stalks of tall green and began ripping out the weeds.

JEREMY'S SONG
CHRISTINE HERBSTRITT

It was to be the summer of celebrations: My grandparent's 50th wedding anniversary, my sister's fall wedding, but first my wedding kicked off the most perfect Memorial Day weekend with clear blue skies and wisps of cotton-ball clouds. Family upon family attended, with so many children we even had a piñata for their entertainment, appropriate in this summer to celebrate family.

Somehow I knew that perfection wasn't meant to last. Just one month later, I came home from work, and started to cry for no reason, sobbing for a solid two hours. My new husband came home and tried to cheer me up. But to no avail. I finally calmed down, but couldn't shake the feeling of dread. Late that night, a phone call from my dad woke me.
"Bad news, Honey."
I replied: "Grandpa died."
"No, worse," He answered "Jeremy."

Jeremy was my 6-year old cousin, the middle child of my youngest uncle. Smart, and mischievous, I pictured his earnest little face with blond slicked-back hair and big brown doe eyes. He and his older brother, Jesse, 8,had been playing in their yard when the inebriated next door neighbor lost control of his car and pinned both boys under it.

My mother answered the phone to the voice of my hysterical aunt.After dispersing my brothers to find my uncle, she, my dad and sister raced to their house. My entire immediate family watched and waited while rescue workers extracted the boys. At one point, Jesse, who suffered severe burns from the exhaust on the lower halves of his legs and would spend the summer in rehab, said. "I don't think my brother's with me anymore."

The two hours I was crying were the two hours the boys had been trapped under the car.

By the end of the weekend's viewing, the small white coffin was filled with trinkets and mementos from the many little cousins who struggled to comprehend it all, as did the rest of us. At the crowded funeral, which is referred to as an angel mass for a young child, a bird somehow made its way into the church through two sets of doors. While sitting in quiet reflection after communion, the bird started to sing. After the closing prayers, as we headed to the grave side, the bird flew out justabove Jeremy's mom's head. All summer long, a red bird would continue to visit her.

Later that summer, Jeremy's 3 year old sister Rachel sat drawing a picture. It showed an adult woman holding the hand of a small boy. "THIS is me when I grow up." She said, pointing to the boy: "That's Jeremy. He's never going to get to grow up."

And in the picture was a red bird.

WHILE MY GUITAR GENTLY WEEPS
(THREE TALES ABOUT GUITARS AND LIFE)
WILLIAM JOHN ROSTRON

1 - THE LAST CHORD

We were a good band. Hell, we were a great band—perhaps, the best band in our part of the city—and it's hard to believe it all started with two stickball bats.

We were ten years old when Gio and I first started to zip spaldeen balls past each other in one-on-one stickball competitions. During winter, we used those same bats to play air guitar along with our favorite records. Gio had the idea to do it with real instruments, and our parents supplied two Silvertone guitars for $20 each from the Sears catalog. By virtue of being silent, the two stickball bats might have sounded better.

One day, Gio arrived excitedly with the news that a friend had taught him how to play the Searchers' "Love Potion #9." Into the night, we played that one song, and Gio started to make-believe that we were in front of an audience.

"Yes, we can play Love Potion #9."

"Oh, you want to hear it again."

"And again."

Imagination can only take you so far when your repertoire is one song. Our night ended when my father threatened to make our two guitars into "$40 worth of kindling" if we didn't stop.

We did stop that night, but it was the beginning of our musical careers together. Eventually, we progressed to electric guitars and added a sensational drummer named Jimmy, who we found while he was using wooden dowels to play the "Wipeout" drum solo in our high school shop class.

We added a lead guitarist and practiced for months, never accepting less than perfection. It paid off. By the following summer, we were playing in clubs in the Village, and then for four thousand people in Central Park. It was all in front of us as we auditioned for a house band job and record contract. That was the beginning of the end.

As the police swarmed into the club, we knew we were in trouble/ The losing band had called the cops on us. Our manager had failed to produce the phony proof he had promised. We knew it was the end of a dream. I quietly slipped off the stage, hoping some of my bandmates could also do so. They couldn't, and Gio winked at my ingenuity when I sidled up the bar and pretended to be a customer. However, I couldn't legally even do that. The raid had been precipitated by us being underage.

I never saw any of the members of the band again. Gio skipped town but not before telling me, "Hey dumbass, the cops never found out about you. Let's keep it that way."

I went on with my life but never ceased wondering what had happened to them. In 2013, I found out that Jimmy Mac had died. Soon after, I located Gio in Florida and spoke to him on the phone. He wouldn't...no, he couldn't answer my questions about that night.

I see him often now that he has moved back to New York. He doesn't know that he moved. He has early-onset dementia. He remembers me because I visit as much as possible. Unfortunately, he remembers very little else.

A few months ago, I brought him to my music room. He quickly wrapped his fingers around the neck of my Fender in position to play the first chord of "Love Potion #9." Then, I picked up another guitar and was ready to join him in the song we first played half a century ago as young, excited teens.

His fingers dropped off the guitar, and as much as he tried, he could not remember where to put them again. I took the guitar and tried to refresh his memory by playing the first few notes of the song that *he* had once taught me.

"That's a nice song. Did that just come out?"

I cried.

I am the only one left to remember our friendship and our band…a band now lost forever in the wind. For Gio and me, that first chord we had ever played together…would now be our last.

2 - DEJA VU ALL OVER AGAIN

I vaguely remember the phrase art imitates life, or is it life imitates art? Hmm? In my case, it was both! While searching for an idea for a particular sequence in my first novel, *Band in the Wind,* I hit upon the idea of using my real-life experience to create the fictional drama for my main character, Johnny Cipp. In the book, the protagonist becomes a bass player in an up-and-coming band. But how could I explain the thought process of someone becoming a bass player? Unless you experience it, it is hard to understand why anyone would subjugate the stardom of being a guitar hero to pound bass notes in the background. So to solve this dilemma, I used my real-life experiences.

In 1965 I was a decent guitar player. I was improving steadily and hoped to achieve so much more. How good could I get? I never found out. While playing on my high school baseball team, an errant pitch crushed my left hand. By the time I recovered, baseball had left me—more ironically, so had music. It became next to impossible to fit my now clumsy fingers onto the frets and strings of a guitar.

One day while trying to solve my problem, I picked up a bass guitar and found that the size and situation of the strings made this relatively easy for me to play. More importantly, I truly enjoyed everything about this unique instrument and its role in a band. I found musical fulfillment with a group that played in Greenwich Village and Central Park.

I had my answer. I merely copied my real-life saga into my novel. The character of Johnny Cipp suffered all I had and dealt with it identically as I did. Why wouldn't he? I created him. I could relive the ritual of soaking my hands in buckets of ice after practicing for hours. I could describe the pain my character experienced by simply retrieving my memories. The true story of a guitar player who became a bass player after an injury in 1965 became the story of a fictional character named Johnny Cipp. It worked well in a whole trilogy of novels. But the story wasn't over.

Writing the books between 2010 and 2020 brought back so many memories that I became enamored with the idea of playing the guitar again. With the onset of the Covid quarantine, I had an excessive amount of free time. A half a century of healing had given me the ability I had lost so long ago. My skills grew as they had never been allowed to during my teen years. My wife bought me a beautiful Fender Stratocaster guitar for Christmas, and the sound quality improved even more. I had rewritten *our* story, both Johnny Cipp's and mine.

In September of 2021, three tumors were found in my lungs. They were just the latest incarnation of a cancer that I had been dealing with for more than a decade. The doctors advised that the only solution would be strong doses of chemotherapy for more than six months. I recovered…but as a side effect, I had lost the use of the tips of my fingers. Whether it was permanent or temporary was undetermined.

I struggled extremely hard to attain the guitar skills I had only recently gained. Many chord changes were filled with clunkers. The more I grew frustrated with playing, the more I looked for a solution, never realizing that it was there right before my eyes—on my bookshelf. The solution of the past was also the solution of the future. I bought myself a new bass guitar and, with a great deal of practice, regained the skills of my youth. I reveled in my ability to lay down the bass tracks for Cream's "Badge" and the Animals' "We Gotta Get Out of This Place." I had come full circle. I had taught my fictional friend Johnny Cipp how to cope with adversity... and now he had taught me.

As Yogi Berra had once said and John Fogerty had written in a song… it was like "Déjà vu all over again."

3 - THE GHOST IN MY GUITAR

"Southy Park" was the poor side of town. Some would have called it the "black part of town," but I was white, and I lived there. My dad had died, and my mom worked hard for what little we had. I didn't mind being there except when the bullies called me a "Southy Turd" and treated me like the second part of that title.

I even chipped in money to support us by searching for old bottles to get the five-cent deposit. Those were the days before recycling laws made plastic bottles a light and cheap goldmine. No, I had to look for rare glass bottles to get my reward. Then again, five cents was worth more in those days. I never realized how bad my life was then, but I knew we were nowhere near the top of the heap.

This is my long way of saying that my bottle-chasing job changed my life—forever. While returning my finds one day, I met Fast Jesse. He was a very old black man who lived on my block but who I had never before had the nerve to talk to. He was skinny and walked and stooped over. He was relatively short, perhaps not much taller than 12-year-old me. A full shock of gray hair set off his dark black skin, and his eyes had a yellow hue that indicated a series of health problems.

Yet his most defining feature was his long, lithe fingers. They alone looked healthy and well-exercised—and I knew why. Fast Jesse played the guitar. Did I say played? He crushed it—his fingers moving like lightning over the frets. The "Fast" part of his name referred to his playing rather than any other part of his existence which was decidedly *slow*-moving. I knew all this because I hid behind the bushes in his front yard many a day and night. I listened intently as he played all types of music, from delta blues to rock and roll. It was rumored that in his youth that he had played the Mississippi Delta juke joints with Smokey Joe Watson and maybe even Robert Johnson.

I would sit there for hours, wishing I could play guitar like him. One day, I found a discarded acoustic guitar in the junk during my bottle-hunting travels. I had saved for weeks to buy strings to put on it. When I got up the nerve, I would peek through his window and see him play. I then would go home and try to recreate what I had seen. It was not going well. The day we met changed all that.

I noticed him immediately but believed he had no idea who I was. He was at the counter paying for some items when I came up from behind him. I noticed that he had about a dozen cans of cat food and used my observation to start a conversation with him.

"Sir, you must have an awful lot of cats?" He looked back at me with a smile but, at first, said nothing. However, I was persistent and repeated my statement.

"No," he mumbled. Then, as he turned, he patted me on the shoulder and shuffled out of the store.

"Mr. Jakes, why didn't he say more to me?" The store owner contemplated long before answering me.

"He don't have no cats."

"But...," I started to say before realizing the answer to my own question. Fast Jesse had little money, and what he had he made stretch by eating cat food.

That night I did more than secretly listen to him play. I took half the dinner my mom prepared for me of chicken legs and po'boy bread and left it on his front porch before knocking and running away. One chicken leg and two fried cornbread balls were not much, but I figured they were better than cat food. The third night I tried this with a small piece of catfish and some greens. Fast Jesse caught me.

"I've done many bad things in my life, but takin' food out of a child's mouth is not one of them," barked Jesse.

"I'm sorry," I started but immediately realized that my act of charity had offended this man's pride— so I improvised. "I thought of it as paying you for the pleasure of listening to your playing," I continued until he cut me off.

"Well, then you owe me back pay because I've been watching you sneak behind that bush over there for more months than I can count."

Okay, so Jesse was sharp-eyed and sharp-minded and had known about me for a long time. I now stood at his doorstep, embarrassed and silent, until he spoke again.

"Now, if you were to throw some food my way now and then, I could think of it as payment for the guitar lessons."

"What lessons?"

"The ones that I'll be giving you."

My mom knew I wanted to play the guitar and thought our arrangement was fantastic. She made our food budget stretch enough that Fast Jesse ate a home-cooked meal every night from that night on.

Sometimes, he even came down the street to our house as our guest. On those nights, he told us stories of the road, of music, and of his life. However, I often brought down his meal and stayed much of the evening, learning everything I could from him.

And so, it went for most of my formative teenage years. Fast Jesse taught me everything he could on his guitar—a Gibson guitar that had seen many hours of playing and could tell a million stories if it could talk. But more than that, the guitar *was* Fast Jesse. When I held it, I could feel all the sweat and blood he had poured into playing it. I could feel that its finish had been polished with the teardrops of a hard life. But most of all, I could understand his love for the music he had played on it.

The years flew by, and I grew as a musician. I was thankful for this beautiful person I had come to think of as a friend. Yet, I knew it could not last forever. Jesse's health was failing, and soon after my seventeenth birthday, I went to see him for the last time. I didn't know it at the time, but he did.

"You take it."

"Take what?" I questioned, but he smiled and nodded at the guitar. I was confused.

"I gotta go."

"Where?" Again, he smiled and shook his head.

"Remember three things. You pray to God, be good to your momma, and take care of this guitar."

I fumbled for something to say but came up with nothing. Why was Jesse saying goodbye? I figured I would humor him. I would take the guitar that night and get some answers the next day.

Fast Jesse died that night. The loss left me with heartbreak—and his guitar. It was a week before I could even pick it up. Every time I looked at it, I remembered that he was gone and immediately laid it back down. Until one day, I didn't.

Slowly, on the tenth night after his death, I lifted it in my arms, put the ancient strap over my shoulder, and tuned it. I started to play. No, it wasn't just me playing. I could feel him in my fingers; I could see his face staring at me and smiling every time I hit a good lick on the strings. He was alive and would always be alive as long as this guitar was played. I somehow knew that.

I went on to have an incredible career in music. I played in bands and sometimes as a solo artist. I made lots of money and lived a life that Fast Jesse had deserved but never gotten. And all those nights playing, I think back fondly. Sometimes, I was in total control, and sometimes I just sat back and felt his heart beating. I could feel all his sweat on the frets as my fingers touched them. I knew that Fast Jesse was in control of the guitar. He was playing the strings through me—just like there was a ghost in my guitar. Fast Jesse would come alive through my hands. I welcomed him.

In all those years of success, I never forgot my roots. I took large amounts of my money and invested in an effort to make the lives of the people of Southy Park just a little bit better. I helped build a church and a rec center and set up a food bank. I don't know if it was all me or if Fast Jesse was still weaving his magic. It didn't matter. It felt good. Eventually, I retired to the place. I could have been in the snooty part of town but didn't want to be. It wasn't real to me.

A few years ago, I met Isaac. I was picking up some groceries at the local convenience store. With a smile, I put a can of cat food in my cart. I did this now and then to remember Fast Jesse and how we met. I have enough money to have someone do my shopping for me, and I certainly would not eat cat food. But Isaac didn't know that. He made the same assumption (incorrectly) that I had made years before about Fast Jesse (correctly).

"Mister, you shouldn't be eatin' that stuff. It's not good for you." I guess kids are not as discreet these days. And no matter how much I tried to persuade him that I wouldn't eat the tin of feline delights, he wouldn't believe me. He took out a wallet and bought me a gigantic sandwich. I noticed that this had taken every bit of money in his possession. I was taken aback by his act of pure unselfishness. I didn't want to tell him it wasn't necessary.

"What's your name?" I asked

"Isaac Beaumont...Junior."

"Well, Isaac Beaumont, Junior, have you ever wanted to learn the guitar?"

"Yeah, I always did, but my family doesn't have enough money for lessons." Was he a guitar wanna-be like me in my youth? This seemed to be too much of a coincidence.

"I think maybe, we can work something out. Let's go see your parents."

Isaac has been my student and my friend for three years now. He is an excellent guitarist and will go a long way—very soon. He just left my house with the guitar, the same one that Fast Jesse gave to me all those years ago. It has served me well, but its time had come to leave. Now my sweat and tears are mingled with those of Fast Jesse. Sadly, after all these years, I will never play it again. It's over. I know it in much the same way that Jesse knew it.

By tomorrow, Isaac will be playing with the ghost in *his* guitar.

ORB OF LIGHT

—Mark Heathcote

If you explore my eyes and light the taper to my soul
you just might-see-my heart explode, my soul implode.
Be left holding an orb of light that's never burned cold
you might be left scorched singed to the eyeballs,

wishing you lit that taper, sooner-all-truth-told.
If you explore my eyes,
and if you light that taper to my soul
there isn't anything in this or the next world I'll withhold.

SENSELESS

WILLIAM JOHN ROSTRON

Chemotherapy has knocked me senseless. Hyperbole? Nope. The treatments indeed took away all five of my senses, rendering me unable to write the books and short stories that I so enjoy working on. However, I think that I am handling the garden variety fatigue, pain, and hair loss with dignity and grace. (Oh, God, where did my beard go?) But the senses, that was a whole new ballgame.

I believe that the first loss I noticed was my hearing. I always have had a slight ringing in my ears because of a tendency to play and listen to very loud music. However, I was surprised when I looked out at the bird feeders on the side of our house and reflected on how very loud the tweeting and screeching were at that moment. Were these birds on steroids? When I moved into the house's interior, I realized the sound had not dissipated. I now understood that it actually was steroids—the massive amount of them coursing through *my* veins and exaggerating the ringing. Still, I think my wife is jealous that I can now hear birds—real or imagined—all day without interruption.

Next up on the hit list was my sense of taste. Gone! I only realized how bad it was when I looked at the box that a delicious-looking pepperoni pizza came in and knew that the cardboard picture of the slice would taste the same as the actual slice sitting before me. This was ironically compounded by the fact that I did NOT completely lose my sense of smell despite the constantly bloody noses. This meant that I could smell the tempting food that I couldn't taste. I began to feel that someone up there was playing a joke on me. I was thrown a crumb when I realized that my total hair loss meant not having to trim those obnoxious nose hairs anymore.

However, the hair loss included my eyelashes, nature's protection against the microscope debris that chronically assaults the eyes. Very soon, the hot compresses, drops, and medication only provided specific periods of definitive sight. My wife and I tried to make the best of it by creating a game where I guessed what was going on during our favorite TV shows. I was mostly wrong.

However, my limited sight was only the beginning. Next to adversely affect my ability to write was the loss of feeling in six of my fingertips, which made using the keyboard almost impossible. A friend suggested that I use a voice-activated program to produce written work. Unfortunately, I had difficulty with painful mouth sores and so held out trying that method. When I gave it a shot, my extreme Queens accent made the entire story appear as if it was written in a cross between Slovakian and Mongolian. But you are reading this, so I guess typing with four fingers works, even if it takes forever.

Senseless, yes, that's me. Well, not actually. I can keep writing as long as I can retain the one sense most vital to me...my sense of humor.

MANDOLIN MAN
MICHAEL P. KUSEN

In a tattered old photo album, I have an old black and white photo of my dad as a young man in the 1930's. He is standing with a broad smile in front of a table displaying an accordion, violin, banjo, mandolin and a harmonica – all the instruments that he could play by ear.

That photo brings back memories of him over the years playing those instruments. I remember him playing polkas on his accordion at family parties. And I remember him strumming a banjo while playing his harmonica that was held in a wired neck holder a'la Bob Dylan.

When I was a teenager and my dad was in his fifties he used to sit in a rocking chair on our porch and strum his old worn mandolin playing a medley of old tunes that were popular in his era and occasionally he would softly sing the lyrics. He even recorded himself once on an old Revere reel to reel tape recorder. I think over time the mandolin became his favorite instrument.

When I was sixteen, I was working on Wall Street as a runner delivering and retrieving stocks and bonds. I was very proud of this new feeling of having my own money in my pocket for the first time in my life. And as my dad's birthday approached in January, I wanted to get him a gift with my new-found income – a gift that would really surprise him and be something special. And so, it was my good fortune to spot a beautiful mandolin prominently displayed in a pawn shop window for a mere twenty-seven dollars (almost half of my 1963 salary). I went into the pawn shop and inspected it – and sure enough it was like brand new.

More than fifty years have passed since I gave my dad that mandolin on his birthday, but I still can recall the look of surprised joy on my dad's face when he opened my present that year. And for the next four years, he played that mandolin until he passed away in 1967. Then the mandolin reverted back to me as a keepsake of my love for my dad. Being devoid of musical talent myself, I hung the mandolin on the wall in my living room. And over the years, I would often look at it and feel a bittersweet sentiment – affectionately remembering my dad.

My dad was gone now for more than twenty years when I was helping my mom do some house cleaning and rearranging. In an old carton in the basement, I found the old Revere tape recorder. I picked it up and put it in a pile to be discarded. But then as I went through another old carton of odds and ends, I found a reel of recording tape that was labeled "Mandolin Man." I froze for a moment recognizing my dad's lettering. Needless to say, I retrieved the old tape recorder, cleaned it up and did some light maintenance on it to make sure it was still functioning.

A short time later I carried the recorder upstairs to the living room and called out to my mom telling her I wanted her to see what I had discovered. She came into the living room and was curious but a little perplexed as I set up the machine and plugged it into the wall outlet.

"Mom, just sit down for a moment. I want you to hear this." I made sure the tape reel was securely in place and switched on the dial to play. The sound of mandolin music stirred in the air and my mother sat transfixed as she heard the voice of her husband singing, *"Baby face, you've got the cutest little baby face. There's not another one that could take your place…"*

I felt a warm sensation as I watched my mother's expression

change from being perplexed to transfixed – she didn't cry but a look came over her face like she was hallucinating in some angelic state.

It's 2013, and I am sitting in a movie theater with my wife watching, *The Book Thief* – a movie she dragged me to after she had read the book and sung its praises to me. The movie was intriguing, and when we left the theater and talked about it, there was something that stuck in my mind like a haunting melody. It was the scene of people huddled in an underground shelter in gloom and desperation and then a man begins to play an accordion and by the magic of music the fear on the faces of the people lightens into a calmness.

That scene got to me, and I couldn't sleep well that evening, but in the morning, something prodded me to go through that old tattered family photo album. And as I turned the pages, I came to the WWII section, and there was my dad in his army uniform standing in the doorway of a building somewhere in war-torn France playing an accordion. My eyes became moist when the thought hit me like a bolt – *my dad did for his comrades what that man in the film had done* – he lifted their spirits with his music.

I'm seventy years old now, having outlived my dad by almost twenty years. And it is time for me to scale down and move into a smaller but more efficient home. And of course, what to do with all the stuff I've accumulated over the years. And then a strange thing happened, the strap on my dad's mandolin (the one I bought for him) broke and the mandolin fell from where it was hanging and landed on the floor. Luckily the mandolin itself was not damaged, only the strap had become brittle. I thought about passing along the mandolin to someone in the family but there were no mandolin aficionados in our family, and I feared it would become a bit of an albatross if someone took it out of obligation to me, because no one could come near the special sentiment of the mandolin that I shared with my father. But a mandolin is meant to be played, and I had kept it as a sentimental decoration long enough. I also had a haunting thought about the mandolin falling from the wall after all these years just as my wife and

I were preparing to downsize and move – was my dad trying to tell me something from the great beyond?

So, I decided to donate it to the Salvation Army – an organization that my dad always thought highly of. It was my hope that the mandolin would find someone who would bring it back to life and strum those waiting strings. I entered the Salvation Army's storefront carrying the mandolin and walked towards the receiving area. But as I rounded a corner towards the counter, I passed a man whose eyes lit up as he stared at the mandolin cradled in my arms. I stopped – call it fate – call it karma – but I felt the presence of my father. I held out the mandolin to the little man with the light in his eyes, "Here," I said. "It's yours – you look like a *Mandolin Man*."

PRECIOUS TIME

–Mark Heathcote

How can we cultivate our precious time?
Midnight and the hour have now long gone.
Let the mother of my heart blow out the candles.
Banish the sunset in its whispery flames.
Choose an amber locket to lock my soul in.
As I sit here alone and watch the moon
feel inside of me an even deeper gloom
the lamp flickers stars fireflies without-names
our tears are just as salty all the same.
Whether-we-lives or died or ever came to be.
How can we cultivate our precious time?
Midnight and the hour have now long gone.

THE ORDINARY MAN AND THE YOUNG PROFESSOR
K. V. RAGHUPATHI

There is a young man in his mid-thirties by the name of Akhilesh who is teaching literature at a university in the temple city of Tirupati. He has devoted himself to intellectual pursuits and has a wide range of knowledge in eastern and western philosophies, literary theories, and aesthetics. He is much adored by the students and much envied by his colleagues for his teaching abilities and scholarship. Nevertheless, he is indifferent to both and has shown the least interest in the praise and the envy. He is known for his avariciousness for reading; so he has spent hours and hours in the university library reading, endlessly oblivious to time and the world. Not a single book has arrived in the library for accession that has escaped his attention; he will grab it from the accessory section and read it before it is given an access number and placed on the racks. Such is his greediness and addiction to knowledge. Wherever he travels, he carries a book and plunges into it when he finds free time.

Thus by reading books, he has become a rationalist, a pure intellectual. Wherever he is found taking part in discussions, he applies logic and wins the debate. He has a knack for persuasion and the power of convincing with his logic and reason. This way, he has won both admirers and enemies.

But not all knowledge is the same to him, nor is any thought as good as any other. He loves a certain type of thinking and disdains and abominates certain types of other thinking. What he loves and reveres is logic, and he is ready to sacrifice for it. In a way, logic has become an integral part of his living, reading, writing, speaking, and argument. It is hard to separate it from his personality. For this, he is nicknamed Logic Akhilesh.

He is not aware, to be sure, of the other sorts of thinking and knowledge for which the sharp intellect becomes useless. What plays a crucial role in such ability is a deep insight by which profound wisdom is acquired. Despite this lack of knowledge, he has not developed any contempt for it. Although he is a free thinker, he is not intolerant of the presence of such knowledge. He is also unaware that such knowledge cannot be gained by reading books. For a long time, he has embraced everything that exists in books and theories with the exception of one single province: the human soul. This ignorance on his part is not a crime, but he considers and calls it a bliss so long as it does not fall under the purview of logic and reason. Call it alien, but the presence of such knowledge cannot be treated as remote antiquity. So he thinks, he speaks, and when traces of such knowledge come to his attention, he becomes restless and feels as if touched by something hostile.

Wheatish in complexion, handsome with strong and regular facial features that look young and appealing, his body sculpted as firm with his back straight, Akhilesh always walked upright as if confident, undefeated, and optimistic. He has never displayed signs of despair in arguments and discussions. His demeanour in all winning and losing situations, unperturbed, he is yet to fall in love nor any woman has ever trapped him. Though he remains the center of attraction in all debates and discussions, women have always admired him for his extraordinary scholarship, but have never tried to become a part of his shadow.

One day it so happened that he felt intensely disillusioned with his knowledge and abstained from the duties in the department without intimating his colleagues in the university or his neighbours and without applying for a formal official leave and disappeared. Nobody knew where he had gone. His two-roomed house in the Nalanda Colony in the temple city is found locked and the neighbours on the inquiry have expressed their ignorance about his whereabouts. A week had passed with no trace.

He left the temple city in despair and was found wandering in the streets of another temple city, Varanasi, a holy city for the Hindus in the north. Varanasi, one of the oldest cities in the world, which makes it rich with cultural heritage, is considered the ultimate pilgrimage spot for Hindus for ages. According to Hindu mythology, it was built by the God Shiva, one of the trinity Gods of Hindus who believe that whoever is graced to die in the city will attain salvation and freedom from the cycle of birth and rebirth. Situated on the crescent-shaped western bank of the river Ganges, it is known as a city of scholars, saints, and sages; it is home to ghats, temples, museums, and many Puranic places. For the seekers of esoteric truth, one's spiritual journey begins with Varanasi.

In Varanasi, Akhilesh, with a brown shoulder bag strapped across his chest, moved aimlessly. The bag contained a towel, a kit, a pair of dresses, and a blanket. He bathed in the Ganges, ate at the pushcart hotels, and slept on one of the stone-stepped Dashashwamedh ghat. One day, while walking, he moved away from the city outskirts and entered the green fields. Crossing the green fields and huge palmyra and coconut trees, he passed into a village studded with hardly a hundred traditional houses, some mud-walled and thatched, some tiled, and a few structured with fragile yet strong exteriors to withstand any kind of harsh weather - all seem to be living close to nature.

A few yards away from the village, beyond the fields, Akhilesh found a small mud walled cottage roofed with a zinc sheet in the shade of palmyra trees. A few feet away from it is found a small brook gurgling through bushes and tree branches with uneven paths on either side. It is occupied by an ordinary man. People in the village called him neurotic. But he did not look so. He always asserted that he was an ordinary man. For this reason, he is forced to live away from the village on the outskirts. Yet four or five people in the village frequently visited him with great reverence for guidance in life, as they saw something singular in his personality.

It is afternoon, and the rays of the sun are falling directly on the village. Passing along the metallic road that cuts through the village, Akhilesh reached the cottage unknowingly. It was not his premeditated thought to meet him. In fact, he knew nothing about the ordinary man living on the outskirts of the village. It was purely accidental. There, he found the ordinary man immersed in his chores. On the first encounter, the ordinary man did not appeal to Akhilesh. Yet, casually, he introduced himself to the ordinary man and awaited the latter's response.

The ordinary man conducted Akhilesh to a garden of flowers. Showing a particular flower, he asked the young man,

"What do you see?"

"I see a flower amidst flowers"

"What do you see?" the ordinary man asked again.

"It is a flower with pink petals," Akhilesh replied undoubtedly.

Not satisfied, the ordinary man once again insisted.

"What do you see?"

"It is a flower with pink petals shooting from a plant."

The ordinary man pursued with intensity.

"What do you see?"

"It is a flower with pink petals emitting a beautiful fragrance that is distinct." Composed, the ordinary man continued with the same question.

"What do you see?"

This time, not losing his temper, Akhilesh replied: "It is a flower named a rose, regarded as the queen of flowers."

Again, the ordinary man demanded a firm reply to his question.

"What do you see?"

Exhausted and upset, Akhilesh did not reply. He kept silent, fearing that the ordinary man would once again bounce with the same question. He stood, instead, in front of the flower, looking at it intently. Now the language of description has gone dry.

The ordinary man did not persist with his question, "What do you see?" He stumbled back to his cottage, leaving Akhilesh in the garden, who kept watching the flower, losing himself in watching. He remained in that state for a long, oblivious to time. It was a great experience, never before has he undergone such an experience in his life. Whatever the experience he had hitherto was purely intellectual;

it was mind-centric. Now, the experience he had was something strange, undecipherable, and distinct from the mind-centric experience. The latter derived from mere reading and gaining scholarship; it was pleasurable. But the experience with the flower was undefinable.

～

Akhilesh, loaded with the undefinable experience, returned to the Dashashwamedh ghat in the city as the sun was slanting in the west. Near the ghat that never sleeps, around 9.30 at night, he had *roti* (made of wheat flour) and *sabji* (vegetable dish) and slept on one of the elevated steps to the rustling waves in the river. The river was full of tranquillity and liveliness. But for Akhilesh, it was disturbing. In sleep, he was confronted with the conversation he had with the ordinary man. The ordinary man was not ordinary, he assured himself.

Morning came with the usual hustle and bustle of the pilgrims flocking to the ghats for the holy bath in the river. Akhilesh too had his morning ablution in the river along with the pilgrims, finished his breakfast, and headed to the cottage in the village as if he had a call from the ordinary man.

On reaching the cottage, he found the ordinary man immersed in his work. Cautiously, he approached him and told him what he had felt about watching the previous day. "It was a beautiful experience that I never had in my life. I lost myself. I did not derive such an experience from reading books. May I know what this experience is?"

The ordinary man had hit Akhilesh on his face, so hard that he started bleeding in the mouth.

Shocked, Akhilesh stood speechless. He never expected such a blow from the ordinary man who went out, leaving him in disbelief to collect some firewood. After an hour, he returned to the cottage, prepared some tea from herbs, and offered a glass to Akhilesh, who was yet to recover from the shocking treatment, without uttering a word about the experience of the blow. As he finished consuming the tea, emboldened, he said, "The blow was terrible. It pained me the whole hour, and I will continue to have it tonight when I get back to the ghat."

On this, the ordinary man transpired nothing but asked, "How is tea?"

Akhilesh sipped the tea from the glass without answering. He could not understand the implication of the blow and the experience. What is the relationship between the experience of the blow and the experience that he had from watching the flower the previous day? He failed to reason out with his bookish knowledge. As he was ruminating over the happening, the ordinary man said that he had some work to do in the woods and walked off with a shovel and an axe. Akhilesh after some time moved out and headed to the city, covering the little swollen mouth with his left palm.

On one of the stone-stepped ghats, he slept in pain after having a small quantity of food. The following day, as he woke up, he noticed the swelling of his left cheek had reduced. As usual, he finished his morning rituals and returned to the cottage with an irresistible desire to meet the ordinary man who seemed extraordinary and enigmatic. On reaching the cottage, he found that the cottage was bolted from the outside. He looked around, but the ordinary man was not found. He might have gone out, he thought and awaited his arrival. After an hour, the ordinary man reached the cottage carrying a bag full of vegetables and fruits, and on seeing Akhilesh, he greeted, to which the latter reciprocated with not much alacrity.

"Have you carried any news from the city?"

"Nothing special. People are, as usual, repeating their actions, performing their day's functions unashamedly."

After a while, he resumed. "You seem to me something special. I am eager to know this part of your living, distinct from that of mine." Akhilesh beseeched the ordinary man who did not respond immediately as his wont. After a few moments of silence between the two, the ordinary man headed towards another village separated by a huge hill, instructing Akhilesh to follow. There was no straight path to reach it. One has, however, to cross the hill to reach the other side. Akhilesh looked at the ordinary man and asked, "How do we reach the other side?"

"I too don't know," replied the ordinary man, admitting his ignorance.

Both of them struggled to climb the hill, facing small pointed rocks, thorny bushes, and pebbles. Each of the two stumbled, tumbled, fell, and bruised their legs. Nonetheless, both reached the other side. They discovered a stream. Because of heavy rains, the stream abutting the hill that was dry throughout the year became buoyant.

"How do we cross this stream?" Akhilesh asked the ordinary man once again.

"I too don't know," came the reply from the tireless, ordinary man.

They waded through the water, pushing the currents, gasping and yelping. Somehow, they reached the other side of the stream.

Fatigued, Akhilesh ceased pursuing the question, but the ordinary man was joyous, enjoying the struggles.

The ordinary man had no affair with the village and both returned to the cottage. "You haven't answered the question I posed," said the embarrassed, young professor.

"I don't remember what you asked," the ordinary man was quick in replying.

"That part of your living is distinct from that of mine. I notice a difference."

The ordinary man did not reply. Instead, he collected an axe from his cottage and headed to the east to cut wood. On seeing a huge muscular tree, he ordered the young Akhilesh to cut it branch by branch.

Akhilesh followed the ordinary man's instructions without resisting. As he started cutting branch after branch, the ordinary man asked, "What is it?" At every persistent question, Akhilesh answered, "tree".

"Does it look like a tree?"

"No."

All branches were slashed. The tree looked bare, like an artifact.

"Does it look like a tree?"

"No…" Akhilesh replied unabashedly.
 Without further waiting for the young man's understanding, the ordinary man collected the slit branches and axe and headed to his cottage.

Notwithstanding the temptation, the young professor has kept visiting the ordinary man day after day with no sign of dissatisfaction but with curiosity. He is unsatisfied with the answers given by the ordinary man, who seems to be blunt in his demeanour.
 Determined to pursue the questions to their logical end, the young professor boldly asked the ordinary man, "Give me a part of the wisdom you have."
 "Who said I have it? I have none. How can I part with it even if I

have?" the ordinary man retorted. After a while, he paced up and down outside his cottage and moved off. As usual, Akhilesh followed him. The ordinary man stopped in front of a tall coconut tree and looked up. The tree bore a cluster of fruits. Pointing at one ripened, the ordinary man asked the young professor to pluck it for him. He is a novice at climbing coconut trees. However, in respect, as instructed, he attempted to climb the tall shooting trunk. Every time he climbed, he slipped and fell. Because of this, he had bruises on his palm and hands.

Disappointed, Akhilesh said, "it is difficult for me to climb and pluck the fruit you wanted. I am not trained in the art of climbing coconut trees."

"Try to bring one back to my cottage." Having ordered, the ordinary man headed towards his cottage. Evening fell, and the stars faintly appeared in the eastern sky. The young professor returned to the cottage, empty-handed. Guilty, yet composed, he stood before the ordinary man expecting the reprimand. Instead, the ordinary was absorbed in his chores.

"I have been coming here to learn from you the art you have acquired over time for which a few people in the village admire you. You are secretly guarding it. I hear your name traveling far and wide from the people who are visiting you in my absence," Akhilesh lamented before the ordinary man.

As usual, the ordinary man did not react to the complaint like a mundane man. Instead, he gave an empty bucket to Akhilesh and asked him to fetch water from a well, two yards away from the cottage, without spilling a drop on the ground.

Accordingly, Akhilesh collected the bucket and trod toward the well. On the way, he was at ease carrying the empty bucket. It took him hardly five minutes to reach the well. The stray dog guarding the cottage and the ordinary man followed him.

After collecting water, Akhilesh turned to the cottage. The bucket was full, and he was constantly reminded of the instruction given by the ordinary man that a drop of water should not spill on the ground.

However he tried, he failed. Hardly had he made a few steps when he tumbled over a piece of stone and fell. The water spilled all over the ground; upset with it, he, however, reached the cottage with an empty bucket.

Akhilesh repeated the action on the firm instruction. Every time he collected and carried the water, it spilled on the ground. Flustered, he made a final attempt but failed. Ashamed, he returned to the cottage with an empty bucket. He could never carry water without spilling a drop on the ground.

The ordinary man said in a punitive tone, "If you cannot carry bucketful water without spilling a drop on the ground, how can you learn the wisdom that you expect from me? It is not about acquiring knowledge from reading books and defeating the enemies in discussions and debates."

Humiliated, Akhilesh returned to the city, ruminating over the incidents.

Once again, the following morning, after consuming a small breakfast, the young professor returned to the cottage. Something irresistible he felt from which he could not escape. The ordinary man is completely different from him. He never sat cross-legged, meditating as numerous mystics are used to. He is like any other human, carrying on his usual chores and paying little attention to the outside world. But it is a puzzle for the young physician that people in the village and far off looked at the ordinary man with veneration.

"What is the secret of your living?" the young professor asked the ordinary man in curiosity marked with anxiety and agitation. "Why do people look at you with reverence even though you deny it? What have these people seen in you and gained or learned from you? What has attracted people so much? But you deny all this. I too don't see anything extraordinary. But somehow, I am attracted to you."

Akhilesh patiently awaited his answers.

As if unheard, the ordinary man was at his chores. But he was humming while doing the chores. He sat, not cross-legged but ordinarily, watching the birds' fun and frolic and listening to their songs, twittering, screams, and squeals. Now and then he turned to the young physician and directed him to look at a pair of particular birds and watch their pranks. Nothing else transpired between them.

After a few long moments, the ordinary man blurted, "As long as you claim you are stupid, the wise claim nothing."

Akhilesh could not understand the implication of the words. He sought further light on his saying.

"The world does not belong to you, nor you to the world. Any discovery is meaningless. It is purely accidental. For this, you need not bloat yourself. You are given an award for that discovery in your world, and not for the creation because you are not the creator, nor the maker. You are a medium by which something that already exists is revealed. That is all." Having said these words, the ordinary man, while walking, pointed out a tiny flower in the shrub. Turning to Akhilesh, he questioned, "Tell me, is it because the flower is there, and you are rewarded for having seen it? Or is it because you are there, therefore, the flower exists, otherwise it is not there?"

It befuddled the young man at his observation. There was no way out for him. To him, the ordinary man seems to be a tough nut to be cracked.

For a couple of days, Akhilesh did not go to the ordinary man, owing to a slight indisposition. On the third day, having recovered from illness, not satisfied with all his reading of esoteric literature, he went to the ordinary man's cottage with confidence and expectation that the latter would offer him a solution for suffering. Though this is a universal problem, it belongs much more to the young professor who has been experiencing it for quite some time on his personal level. He has tried all means to overcome his suffering but failed.

Now, he is with the ordinary man who narrated a beautiful story with a lot of humour and fun. Having narrated the story, the ordinary man himself started laughing. He went on laughing. Infected by his laughter, Akhilesh too joined and laughed. But there seemed no end to the laughter. The ordinary man went on laughing and laughing so much that at one point, he had to be served with water to overcome his hiccups. Akhilesh was no match to the ordinary man's capacity to laugh. He got exhausted. He could no longer laugh; he felt he had lost his lung power. Feeling ashamed that he was no match for the ordinary man's capacity to laugh, the young man got up, bowed, walked out, and wandered for some time around the cottage to get back to his normal senses.

He returned to the cottage and found the ordinary man too was in normal senses. There was no laughter. The atmosphere seemed to be charged with serenity.

At this point, Akhilesh quoted from several texts that he had read before the ordinary man to prove his scholarship as well as to substantiate his point of argument in disproving the practice of spirituality. It was a clever strategy adopted by Akhilesh to defeat the ordinary man in terms of having read many books. The ordinary man is also a learned person, but his learning is entirely different from that of Akhilesh whose scholarship and argument are based on reason and logically derived from excessive reading. While the ordinary man's wisdom has derived from his living experiences.

The ordinary man quietly listened to Akhilesh. He allowed the latter to exhaust himself completely. There was no other way for him to counter.

Akhilesh fell silent, speechless after displaying his scholarship. He awaited the ordinary man to respond. But, much to his consternation, there was no response from the ordinary man who got up and went inside his cottage and brought the vessels that he constantly used for his chores. He collected a little fine sieved sand and mixed it with lime and applied it to the vessels. He rubbed the vessels, both inside and outside, and washed them with water. The vessels started shining in the sunlight.

"Do you clean the vessels every day?" asked Akhilesh in askance.

"Yes, the vessels may develop stains if I don't wash them every day. I want the vessels to be clean and shining so that the food prepared using them will be hygienic."

The ordinary man's life is an enigma. It is beyond Akhilesh's knowledge of understanding acquired from reading books. He does not seem to distinguish between the knowledge that comes from books and the wisdom that arises from living and observing. The former makes one restless as there is no end to meeting the pleasures unsatisfied, while the latter creates serenity in one's life. He is unable to resolve the confusion that arose from his frequent meeting with the ordinary man. Nevertheless, he began learning a great deal from his interactions with the ordinary man. So he continued his pursuits.

Back in the cottage, Akhilesh said with alacrity, "I have a deep yearning to learn and experience Truth."

"Who said there is Truth?" the ordinary man retorted. "I know nothing of it. If you know, tell me what it is, how it is to be sought."

"Saints and sages have testified to it by their experience. I have read."

"How can you establish Truth if there is one such? I know this body and this mind. Beyond these two, I know nothing. So I take care of these two. I am less worried about that which lies beyond this body and mind. I am worried about the awareness of this body and mind, and I know nothing about the awareness outside of me."

Spellbound, Akhilesh did not pursue the question/s but did not move from there. The ordinary man went out to perform his chores. After a few minutes, he returned to the cottage.

"Where exactly do I go from here?" Akhilesh asked.

"You go nowhere from here," replied the ordinary man, hanging the clothes outside the cottage. "The sun goes nowhere." Pointing at it, he said. "It has been there forever, emitting the light, and it lightens the whole universe. The mountain does not move, but birds, animals, and humans go there."

Akhilesh couldn't understand the implication. He stood before the ordinary man in askance, as if expecting more light on what the latter had said cryptically and metaphorically. "All pursuits and running here and there to deliver the goods, in anticipation of changing the outside, is a mirage." Having said that, the ordinary man was immersed in his chores without caring how Akhilesh would react. He thought his frequent visits and meetings with the former would serve no purpose.

"Why do I care if you don't come? Who asked you to come here? Did I?" The ordinary man was quick in his reply when the young man expressed his wilful desire to leave. "The mountain would never move. The mountain is wisdom."

"You are keeping aloof." The young man said, despondently. "The mountain would not move."

"The society has become corrupt."

"The mountain would not move."

"Society needs you."

"The mountain would not move."

"Man is dying…"

"The mountain would not move."

"Hinduism and Buddhism talk so much about meditation, the way to attain self realization. Teach me at least how to meditate." Akhilesh asked the ordinary man.

"Show me the self. Where is it? Then we can talk about meditation."

"It is practiced in the entire world."

"I don't know." The ordinary man replied in full confidence.
"What is the way?"
"I don't know"
"You are bluffing."
"The sun is going behind the hills."
"Are you misleading?"
"The full moon is rising with splendour and glory."
"Are you misdirecting?"
"The evening star is visible in the twilight sky."
"You are selfish!" The young professor, notwithstanding, uttered offensively.
"The birds are roosting," said the ordinary man joyously.

Akhilesh, disappointed and defeated, rose, came out and headed back to the city without further debating. The ordinary man cared little. As usual, he sat on a piece of rock outside his cottage and watched the beetles rolling mud balls. For Akhilesh, he seems to be incorrigible.

The ordinary man has never experienced pain in his life! Nobody has ever harmed him, nor has he inflicted torture on himself. It is strange and incredible for Akhilesh that the ordinary man has never undergone any bad experience in his life that would have made him suffer a lot.

One day, Akhilesh contrived a plan. He collected a couple of ruffians in the city and went to the cottage in the dead of night when the whole village was asleep. He, along with the two ruffians, entered the cottage through the front door, which was always open, and found the ordinary man was asleep. He was in his deep sleep, and almost lost his body's consciousness. Like deadwood, he lay there.

All three tied him tightly to the cot with a rope, pinning both the hands and the feet. But the ordinary man never awoke. He was in his deep sleep. There was nothing to steal from his cottage. He has a few sundry things that have no value.

The next morning, Akhilesh walked into the cottage and found the ordinary man was attending to his usual chores. There was no sign of pain or restlessness on his face. He was happy, smiling.

Dumbfounded, Akhilesh stood for a few moments and later asked the ordinary man about his welfare, who replied stoically that he was all right, and there was no reference to the previous night's incident. Unbelievable for Akhilesh how this ordinary man has acquired that sense of equanimity in his life. He felt guilty but did not reveal the truth that he had hatched the plot. Without returning to the city, he stayed back in the cottage to pursue the path of learning.

He turned to the ordinary man and asked, "teach me what mindfulness is."

"Where is mind?"

Akhilesh showed, pointing his finger at his head.

"Bring it here. I want to see it."

"How can I?"

"Then don't talk about it."

After a long pause, Akhilesh resumed. "How can I know it? How can I make it 'fullness'?"

"First, bring it here. Then I can talk about its fullness."

"But..." Akhilesh uttered, and stopped, incapable of pursuing further.

"If you make it 'fullness', there is no mind. If there is a mind, there is no fullness," the ordinary man said with zeal.

"How can I understand this?"

"If there is fullness, there is little chance to create. If there is a mind, there is little chance to stop the activity. Which one do you choose? Choosing is a bad act. Just be."

Akhilesh was perplexed at the seemingly complex statement.

"When you do not know how to value what is given to you, all pursuits are meaningless," said the ordinary man in an extraordinary way.

"Give me the clarity." Akhilesh insisted.

"Hold on to what you have. If you try for the 'other', you will lose that which you have. That which is given is more precious than that which is not given or that which is yet to happen, or that which is acquired by effort. That which you have at this moment is more valuable than that which you do not have. By the time you realize the value of that which is given to you, you have missed everything. There is no point in regretting it."

Even before the coop was shut, all cocks and hens had fled. The old man sat on a mound and brooded nothing.

Akhilesh sat facing him, uttering nothing.

"To be one with what you are doing and not with 'you' is real action," said the ordinary man when the young man said, "I have completed the work you have assigned to me."

"After incubating the eggs, the mother bird feeds the chicks. It is an act of *dharma*. The mother bird is living by herself; the chicks are learning to survive. It is not a ritual. It is not an act of pride. While hunting the prey, the mother bird notices that her talons are red with blood. Thank God. It's only the blood of the prey, the mother's talons are intact! You should have this much awareness of the little things you do in your life."

Having uttered these words, the ordinary man shared tea with the young man. "Is everything fine?"

"It is okay. I am not committing a crime. I take it easy."

"I am sick and tired of having met you so many times. Can I go now?"

"Did I ask you to meet me? No female bird has ever invited a male bird for mating. But it is happening. The female bird mates with the male bird on no invitation. There is no choice. But it is happening."

"I cannot bet you for what you have given me," said the young man in gratitude.

"Sorry, I cannot give you for what you have learned nothing from me," said the ordinary man audaciously but marked with humility.

The young man was perplexed at this. Yet, he repeated, "Can I go now?"

"Which moves, the body or the mind? Nothing moves, but everything happens. You are a fool," replied the ordinary man swiftly. After a few moments of pressing silence, he resumed, "There is nothing you need to worry about in this creation. Everything is taken care of in nature. You won't have anything to do with the mad race everyone else is in."

Akhilesh was not convinced. He was still skeptical. How could one live without doing anything in the world? He thought. But looking at the way the ordinary man was living in a small cottage, away from the hustle and bustle of life in towns and cities, Akhilesh seemed to have been confused.

"This is a very childish way of thinking; I cannot live in this world. Damn it." The ordinary man continued. "Why are you here? Get lost in the world. I can hardly be useful to you." He commanded Akhilesh in anger.

The young man, upon listening to the ordinary man's command, wanted to leave, but an irresistible attraction made him hesitant. However, conceding that the ordinary man was in a fit of emotion, Akhilesh decided to leave. But even before he retreated, the ordinary man slipped into his cottage and reclined on the bare floor.

"The truth is that you are fundamentally discontent with what you have and what you don't have. That is, you are running here and there seeking comfort," said the ordinary man in confrontation with the young man.

"But I am not seeking comfort. I am seeking learning that can release me from discontentment and disillusionment."

"Then, go and die. Commit suicide," said the ordinary man angrily.

"That happens in depression. But I am not in depression to commit suicide," replied the young man audaciously.

"Growing oneself physically and materially is easier than not growing. Not growing with oneself is painful and suffocating. Therefore, the mad race."

"How can I take the plight into myself?"

Just then, the ordinary man saw a snake slithering into the water to reach the other side. The young man thought that the water in the pond would suck the snake. But the snake reached the other side and slid into thick shrubs and creepers.

"You cannot be perfect, even the creation is perfectly imperfect and imperfectly perfect," said the ordinary man to Akhilesh who reacted quickly saying, "But you seemed to be perfect with the creation."

"I am evolving to be... Flowers blossom even if you do not admire them. Birds sing even if you do not lend your ears. The tiger hunts even if you stop it."

"You are unique."

"Running water does not go back."

"You are an incorrigible nut to be cracked."

"Waves do not rise like tides."

"Why don't you show a way to the world?"

"Sucked water in the sand cannot be reduced."

"Can I live with you permanently? Take me as your disciple."

"I am a second-hand *guru* for you. I am of little use to you. Get lost in the world. You are a lone traveller."

"To me, you seem to be an enlightened Yogi," said Akhilesh notwithstanding the temptation.

"If you encounter a Yogi, kill him at once," responded the ordinary man instantly. He knew he was speaking consciously and responsibly. "Kill him inwardly."

"How can I kill the enlightened Yogis? They are the real masters. They guide humanity. They can lighten our path, remove obstacles."

"Any clinging is imitation. You can hardly bring your sense of originality. You can hardly strive. You can hardly realize the goal. You can remain a follower of such masters. By following, you can show off. The enlightened Yogi is the biggest obstacle in your journey. Create your own path and tread it. While passing, erase the footprints so that such footprints left behind will not be used by anyone. Ultimately, you are unique in your own way." Having uttered these profound words, he paused and peered around. After a few long moments, he resumed, "The only way to learn how to run is to run. There is no other way. No training institute can teach you how to run unless you are participating in a contest. Nor should you look for such a thing in the world. Don't make yourself a fool. Don't go to anyone to learn it. Learn it by yourself." Later, he ordered Akhilesh to prepare the broth.

Akhilesh did not know how to prepare the broth. But he had to prepare for the ordinary man who wanted it instantly. Akhilesh, notwithstanding his inexperience and little knowledge, prepared it and brought it in a bowl, and placed it before the ordinary man who after sipping once threw it consciously. The bowl rolled and stood upside down, spilling broth all along creating multiple designs on the floor.

Akhilesh once again prepared broth and brought it fresh in a bowl. This time the ordinary man got up from the cot and pretended to pick up a roller from a stand. He fell on the bowl and it once again spilled broth on the floor. Akhilesh, not irritated, once again made broth, but this time while carrying the bow his toes tripped and fell across. He held the empty bowl tightly, while the broth spilled on the floor.

The fourth time, Akhilesh prepared broth, fresh, and placed it once again before the ordinary man who sipped and complained about its taste.

The fifth time, Akhilesh once again prepared the broth, fresh, brought it, and placed it before the cot. Just then, the ordinary man had gone out to attend calls of nature. As he returned, he noticed the cat was sipping the broth.

The sixth time, Akhilesh prepared the broth and carefully brought it, and handed it to the ordinary man who sipped slowly and commented nothing about the taste but simply smiled. The young man felt pleased with this and went out, celebrating his success.

The ordinary man went out on fieldwork. The dissatisfied Akhilesh accompanied him like a chick to its mother. After a day's work in the fields, the ordinary man rested a while on a piece of rock near a pond. He collected a stone and threw it in the pond, and its water rustled. The ordinary man asked the young man, "can you see your image?"

"I can see, but it is not steady and not clear."

After a while, the rustles created by the stone settled. Now, the pond looked as if covered with a glass sheet.

"Can you see your image?"

"Yes. It is clear and perfect." Akhilesh understood the subtle meaning of what the ordinary man was trying to drive. "The problem is how to keep me, like the pond, free from rustles."

"Keep watching. Be an endless spectator in the creation. You can do nothing beyond this." Having said these words, which seemed to be horrifying to Akhilesh, the ordinary man quietly left the cottage and disappeared into the fields. Akhilesh waited long for his return, but in vain. The ordinary man's signs of his return to the cottage did not take place, though the dusk had fallen. Disappointed and gloomy, Akhilesh retraced his own way and left for the city.

∼

Back in the city, Akhilesh had his food and slept on one of the stone-stepped ghats. He woke up to the pilgrims' movements in the early hours. It was four in the morning. After bathing in the mellifluous river Ganges that runs through the city, he had hot *roti* and *sabji* and tea in a mud cup in the city. He returned to the river banks and walked all along the ghats, watching numerous boats with pilgrims and tourists. It was nine in the morning. The sun peeled off the mist over the river, and the buoyant waves suckled the light as the birds flew circling and criss crossing over its chest. The river looked pleasant, bubbling with life on the ghats.

He reached the southernmost Assi ghat and sat on one of the steps in the shade of a peepal tree far away from the people and contemplated watching the clogged plastic bags, clothes, and photo frames thrown by the pilgrims being carried by the waves. Especially, he ruminated over the ordinary man's crisp, quick, and epigrammatic responses that carried profound philosophy and meaning.

More than a month has passed since Akhilesh arrived in the city. He rarely remembered his university and his colleagues at Tirupati as he was immersed in his meetings with the ordinary man. The interactions were now over. He brooded a great deal on his condition. He felt he was all right. He did not go insane. If that were so, it is better to die. The reason is necessary, but the knowledge of the ordinary man is equally important to live in the world. It occurred to him, and perhaps this was a miracle for him. Over a month, his encounters with the ordinary man were accidental. He never thought and dreamt that it would happen. There was no such thing as magic or sorcery, and the ordinary man was not a wizard. It helped him to slow transformation in him.

He spent a couple of days in the city on the ghats. There was no purpose if he had stayed further. He felt unwell and uneasy. He wanted to leave, and he left the city for Tirupati on his own as he came to Varanasi. From one holy city to another holy city, a journey in transformation of himself, from the state of the arrogance of bookish knowledge to a state of shedding it and acquiring new knowledge of self-transformation.

Back at the university and the department, his appearance has given a big surprise and shock to everyone who gathered around him in disbelief and inquired about his welfare and his whereabouts for forty days. Akhilesh stood smiling without uttering a word. After a few long moments, he walked straight to Professor Naveen Chandra's room. He, in his fifties, is now heading the department. He holds a Ph.D. from the University of Wales with a specialization in modern British drama. On seeing Akhilesh, he was nonplussed staring at him. Nothing has transpired between the two except exchanging salutations and brief enquiries about health. There was no reference to his absence. Without waiting further, Akhilesh removed a sealed cover from his shoulder bag and placed it on the table.

"What is it?" The Head asked in surprise and doubt, holding it in his hands as if weighing it.

"Do not open it until I move out of the department. Forward it to the Registrar of the university." Akhilesh said coolly. Professor Naveen's suspicion grew, nevertheless. No sooner has Akhilesh placed the sealed cover than he walked out upright as Professor Naveen, dumbfounded, stood rising from the chair in disbelief and strode fast without transmitting a word to his colleagues, who have gathered in great excitement and relief amid suspicious whisperings. Reaching the main gate of the campus, he vanished like a wisp of cloud as his colleagues stood watching in an utter daze.

ABOUT THE AUTHORS

SHAI AFSAI

Shai Afsai lives in Providence, Rhode Island. Enough said.

MARK ANDREW HEATHCOTE

Mark Andrew Heathcote is adult learning difficulties support worker. He has poems published in journals, magazines, and anthologies both online and in print. He resides in the UK and is from Manchester. Mark is the author of "In Perpetuity" and "Back on Earth," two books of poems published by Creative Talents Unleashed.

CHRISTINE HERBSTRITT

Wife and mother to three daughters, Christine's previous lives include nonprofit management, grant writing and fund development. She currently is employed at a Senior Care Facility, which provides her a plethora of stories. She has had a handful of her creative writings published. Among her other creative endeavors include original hand needle felting and quilting.

MARYANNE J. KANE, PHD

Kane has thirteen publications: seven articles in Newsweek Magazine on education reform, two articles in The Catholic Reporter on pain and suffering, and one article in CatholicPhilly.com on mother-daughter bonding. She has two Flash Fiction pieces in Borrowed Solace (Spring, 2019) and one Flash Fiction piece in Coffin Bell (Summer, 2019). Her first novel, Tattletales from School - Bullying in the 1960s, enjoyed publication with Words Take Flight, August 2022. Kane's Ph.D. is in research in Music Education from Temple University with 30 plus years of teaching experience in private and public schools in Philadelphia and Delaware County. When she's not at her desk writing, she's a volunteer violinist at area churches.

MICHAEL P. KUSEN

Michael P. Kusen is an author illustrator who has created seven instructional chess books and four poetry chap books. He has also published essays, news articles and a family history. His poems and cover art have appeared in The Performance Poets Annual Anthology. Three of his poetry volumes, including children's Chess Poems, are in the Poets House library collection in Manhattan. Michael is currently working on a collection of short stories and essays — he is also juggling several background projects including illustrated poems and assemblage art. mqsen@aol.com

SALLY QUON

Sally Quon is a dirt-road diva and teller of tales, living in the Okanagan. She has been shortlisted for Vallum Magazine's Chapbook Prize two consecutive years and is an associate member of the League of Canadian Poets. Her work has been published in numerous anthologies including Chicken Soup for the Soul—the Forgiveness Fix, BIG, Straightening Her Crown, and Worth More Standing. Her personal blog, https://featherstone-creative.com is where she posts her backcountry adventures and photos.

K. V. RAGHUPATHI

A former academic, poet, short story writer, novelist, critic, and book reviewer, he has so far published thirteen collections of poetry, two short story collections, and two novels, and edited eight critical works and is widely published and anthologized. His poems and short stories have been featured in various online and print journals. Currently, he lives in Tirupati and he can be reached at drkvraghupathi9@gmail.com.

WILLIAM JOHN ROSTRON

William John Rostron's books have a readership that spans five continents and all fifty states. His series of novels steeped in the late 20th and early 21st centuries' music and culture, Band in the Wind, Sound of Redemption, and Brotherhood of Forever, have received critical acclaim from Writers Digest, the Online Book Club Review, and have consistently received Amazon ratings of 4.5 out of 5, or higher. He recently added to this series with The Other Side of the Wind, a book that may be read either independently of the series or in addition to it. He has published over three dozen short stories in anthologies, five receiving awards from Writers Digest this year. Most of these pieces appear in his short story compilation, A Flamingo Under the Carousel. Five of his pieces have been produced on the New York stage and taped. They are available for viewing on the author's website. www.WilliamJohnRostron.com

Born and raised in Queens, NY, William John Rostron now splits his time between his home on Long Island and traveling the country in his Tiffin motorhome. He is busy completing a bucket list of travel adventures when not writing. In the past 18 years, he and his wife, Marilyn, have traveled 140,000 miles. These journeys have taken them to the 48 contiguous states, 133 national parks, all 30 major league baseball stadiums, 154 cities and towns, two Canadian provinces, and various unusual experiences and locations. Many of these locations have served as backgrounds for his books.

He is presently working on a second book of short stories tentatively titled T-Rex Stole My Computer.

www.WilliamJohnRostron.com

JIM TRITTEN

Jim Tritten is a retired Navy carrier pilot living in a small village in New Mexico with his Danish author/artist wife and two cats.

ALSO FROM THE RED PENGUIN COLLECTION

FICTION

What Lies Beyond – Sci-Fi Stories of the Future
I Can't Find My Flashlight – Contemporary Campfire Stories
A Heart Full of Love – A Collection of Romantic Short Stories
Behind Closed Doors – A Mystery Anthology
Once Upon A Time… – A Fairy Tale Anthology
Ernest Lived …and other Historical Fiction Short Stories
Until Dawn – A Supernatural Anthology
Treat-or-Trick – Halloween Horror Stories
Pets On the Prowl – An Animal Mystery Anthology
My Robot & Me – A Not-So Fiction Anthology

POETRY

'Tis The Seasons – Poems to Lift Your Holiday Spirits
the flower shop on the corner – A Spring Poetry Anthology
the ocean waves – A Summer Poetry Anthology
the leaves fall – An Autumnal Poetry Anthology
Proud to Be – A Pride Poetry Collection
Words for the Earth – A Poetry Project
Dear You – Poems Through the Heart

THE STAND OUT SERIES

Stand Out – The Best of The Red Penguin Collection, Vol. 1
Stand Out – The Best of The Red Penguin Collection, Vol. 2

www.ingramcontent.com/pod-product-compliance
Lightning Source LLC
Chambersburg PA
CBHW060407080526
44583CB00012B/498